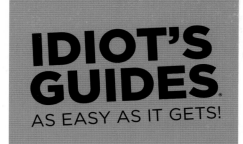

IDIOT'S GUIDES
AS EASY AS IT GETS!

W9-BNX-544

Yoga

by Sarah Herrington

Photography by Kotaro Kawashima

ALPHA

A member of Penguin Group (USA) Inc.

ALPHA BOOKS

Published by Penguin Group (USA) Inc.

Penguin Group (USA) Inc., 375 Hudson Street, New York, New York 10014, USA • Penguin Group (Canada), 90 Eglinton Avenue East, Suite 700, Toronto, Ontario M4P 2Y3, Canada (a division of Pearson Penguin Canada Inc.) • Penguin Books Ltd., 80 Strand, London WC2R 0RL, England • Penguin Ireland, 25 St. Stephen's Green, Dublin 2, Ireland (a division of Penguin Books Ltd.) • Penguin Group (Australia), 250 Camberwell Road, Camberwell, Victoria 3124, Australia (a division of Pearson Australia Group Pty. Ltd.) • Penguin Books India Pvt. Ltd., 11 Community Centre, Panchsheel Park, New Delhi—110 017, India • Penguin Group (NZ), 67 Apollo Drive, Rosedale, North Shore, Auckland 1311, New Zealand (a division of Pearson New Zealand Ltd.) • Penguin Books (South Africa) (Pty.) Ltd., 24 Sturdee Avenue, Rosebank, Johannesburg 2196, South Africa • Penguin Books Ltd., Registered Offices: 80 Strand, London WC2R 0RL, England

International Standard Book Number: 978-1-61564-420-9
Library of Congress Catalog Card Number: 2013940221

15   14   13   8   7   6   5   4   3   2   1

Interpretation of the printing code: The rightmost number of the first series of numbers is the year of the book's printing; the rightmost number of the second series of numbers is the number of the book's printing. For example, a printing code of 13-1 shows that the first printing occurred in 2013.

Note: This publication contains the opinions and ideas of its author. It is intended to provide helpful and informative material on the subject matter covered. It is sold with the understanding that the author and publisher are not engaged in rendering professional services in the book. If the reader requires personal assistance or advice, a competent professional should be consulted. The author and publisher specifically disclaim any responsibility for any liability, loss, or risk, personal or otherwise, which is incurred as a consequence, directly or indirectly, of the use and application of any of the contents of this book.

Most Alpha books are available at special quantity discounts for bulk purchases for sales promotions, premiums, fund-raising, or educational use. Special books, or book excerpts, can also be created to fit specific needs. For details, write: Special Markets, Alpha Books, 375 Hudson Street, New York, NY 10014.

Trademarks: All terms mentioned in this book that are known to be or are suspected of being trademarks or service marks have been appropriately capitalized. Alpha Books and Penguin Group (USA) Inc. cannot attest to the accuracy of this information. Use of a term in this book should not be regarded as affecting the validity of any trademark or service mark.

Publisher: *Mike Sanders*

Executive Managing Editor: *Billy Fields*

Acquisitions Editor: *Karyn Gerhard*

Development Editor/Proofreader: *Megan Douglass*

Production Editor: *Jana M. Stefanciosa*

Cover/Book Designer: *Rebecca Batchelor*

Indexer: *Johnna VanHoose Dinse*

Contents

Dedication

To my parents, for the strong roots.

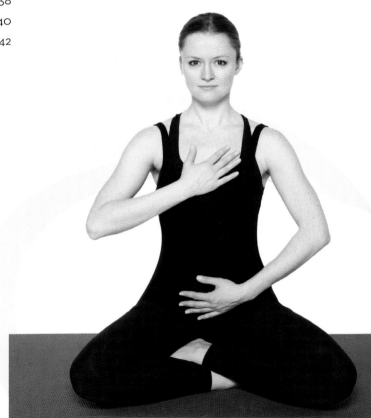

Introduction

Yoga is 99% practice and 1% theory.
—Pattabhi Jois

My first true yoga class was an hilarious experiment. I had just graduated from college when my roommate at the time came across some free passes to a local studio. We decided to take a Saturday afternoon to try a class together. However, we accidentally walked into an "advanced-intermediate" class as total beginners. We were astounded by the deep breaths, focus, and physical feats happening around us. As legs went up into the air in headstands, I remember looking over at my friend and cracking up. We had no idea what we'd gotten ourselves into! We kept giggling as we tried everything from Downward Facing Dog to Tree Pose for the first time. But honestly, we still had a blast. We worked up a sweat and a healthy curiosity, even if we did feel fidgety during the long quiet of seated meditation after Corpse Pose.

Thinking back, both of us could have used a book like this before class. It would have been a comfort to have understood some of the poses and techniques before hitting the mat with a room full of students.

But luckily, even without knowing much about the practice I noticed some strong hints that this was a Good Thing. After class my body felt relaxed and strong. My mind felt calm yet focused. My spirits were lifted; I felt happy. I remember walking down 5th Avenue with my friend afterward and really noticing things I hadn't on the walk there. Before class I'd been rushing with a stressed-out mind. After class I felt more attentive. I remember feeling full of creative energy and having the urge to go home and write, which I did. These feelings offered many clues to the joy and power of yoga practice.

Is Yoga For Me?

Yoga is a word that means "union" or "yoke" in Sanskrit and is a tradition that links body, mind, breath, and spirit. Though the roots of yoga are ancient—and were first written, taught, and expressed in India where Hinduism and Buddhist thought thrived—yoga is a practice for anyone of any age, background, belief system, or body type. The best time to practice yoga is always now. You can start no matter where you are, or what is happening in your body and life. You don't have to be flexible or able to stand on your head to try yoga. As long as you are breathing there's some yoga you can do, and benefit greatly from.

Yoga will help your body become more balanced, improving flexibility and strength in all parts of the body. You will find yourself becoming more fit and physically well through yoga practices, no matter your age or abilities. Working mindfully with your body over time, you begin to tune in and sense what you need. The deep focus of yoga can be a true moving meditation, guiding your mind to clarity and calm. The effects of this mind state begin to spill over into daily life, adding peace and efficiency to actions, even in a multitasking world. The breath and movements of a yoga class can elevate your spirits, leading you to feel happy and well. Many, including myself, view yoga as a wonderful spiritual practice; a way to connect with gratitude and devotion to the divine, to the world around us, and to our deepest selves. No matter what you are looking for through yoga you're bound to receive it, and more. Yoga is a playground for learning.

What Kind of Yoga Should I Do?

There are many types of yoga, and many yoga practices. That's good news. If you find you don't love one yoga class, you can try another in a different style! You may even find that different styles of yoga resonate with you at different times in your life. The poses and practices in this book primarily fall under the umbrellas of *Hatha*, *Vinyasa*, and Power yoga. But you will find a description of different yoga styles and names you may encounter—such as *Bhakti* (devotional) yoga and Restorative (restful) yoga—in the glossary of this book.

You will hear yoga referred to as a "practice." This is an important word. You cannot simply read about yoga and receive all the benefits. My hope is that this book serves as an invitation to *try*! And since it's a practice, you get to try and try again. You don't have to be perfect. It's not about making the best looking shape in a pose, but about the sincerity of your efforts. By showing up to your yoga mat regularly you can really get to know yourself, cultivate peace, and begin to shift your body and life from the inside out. Having a consistent practice can be an anchor in a world full of change.

You are your own best teacher. Though I am here to guide you and share poses, breathing exercises, and even tools for mindful living, as you try things yourself I urge you to pay attention to how they affect you. As you go you'll form a relationship with your body and your self and will become more aware of how things feel to you. You'll become better friends with your own mind and body. Listen to your own inner wisdom. Take the guidance of this book and teachers, but know that you have much wisdom within.

I'm so grateful to share the beautiful and fun practices of yoga with you. Whether you're brand new to yoga or an old pro, I hope this book will help you, find health, wellness, and peace—and that, when you do hit the mat in a class, your only laughter will be of joy.

> *Yoga is the state where you are missing nothing.*
> —Shri Brahmananda Sarasvati

Acknowledgments

It truly takes a community to make a book; I am so grateful to the following rockstar folks for helping contribute to *Idiot's Guides: Yoga*!

First, thanks go to the entire publishing team. Much gratitude to my fabulous acquisitions editor Karyn Gerhard, without whose vision and guidance this book would not be. Many thanks also go to our thorough development editor Megan Douglass and to our gifted designer Becky Batchelor. Gratitude also to wonderful publisher Mike Sanders. I feel blessed to have been part of such a team!

Kotaro Kawashima, thank you for the gift of your fantastic photography in this book. And a big shout-out to my wonderful yoga models Jennifer Link, Sara Schwartz, and Steve Chan—you were all a joy. Thanks also to Carol Tessitore for helping me edit some additional shots. It was so fun to work with you all, and I can truly feel your love for yoga in the beauty and joy of these images.

A special thanks to Yoga to the People for your community during this shoot and for the sharing of props! You are family. Speaking of, thank you to my family and friends for providing support as I worked on this project—in particular, Ashley Inguanta for being a writing friend and cheerleader.

And, as always, thank you to my own yoga teachers past, present, and future.

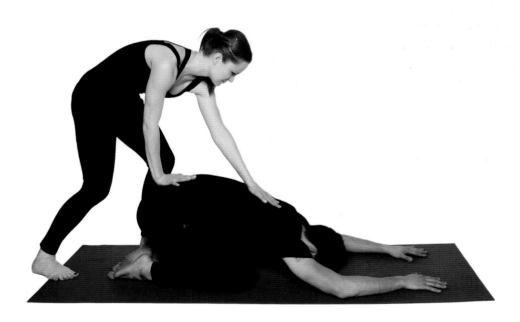

GETTING STARTED

Whatever you can do, or dream you can, begin it. Boldness has genius, power, and magic in it.

–Goethe

BEFORE YOU BEGIN

How to Use This Book

This book is designed to make the exploration of yoga easy and, hopefully, fun! In Part 1, you'll learn about some of the common tools of the practice. From there, you'll be introduced to breathing exercises. Breath work is a big part of yoga. You can try the breathing on its own here, and then have these techniques available to use during poses. It is the mindful use of breath that brings the transformative power of yoga to life.

In Part 2, we'll learn poses one at a time and in-depth. Take the time to try each pose, paying attention not just to your final shape but to how you move in and out of postures. The poses are grouped by type, though it's important to note there is a lot of overlap in these labels. Poses are separated into the following qualities: flexibility, balance, strength, grounding, and restorative. If you're looking to work on your flexibility, you can start there. If you need some deep rest, you can flip to the restorative section. But you'll quickly see all poses give the gift of many qualities at once!

The poses are assigned a skill level from 1 to 5. Please note that this is meant as a guide; the levels are subjective. (There were no number levels in the ancient yoga texts!) A level 1 pose is safe, solid, and accessible for a first-time yogi. Level 3 achieves mid-level difficulty in terms of balance, strength, and concentration required. Level 5 is the most advanced. As always, listen to your body and learn which poses are the most accessible and which are the most challenging for you.

In Part 3, we'll explore advanced variations of the poses we learned together in Part 2, as well as some new and more advanced poses. We'll learn about the 8 Limbs of Yoga and the philosophical and spiritual background of yoga, as well as the concept of mindful eating. We'll also go beyond poses to learn about mudras (energy locks; hand gestures), mantras (sound work), chakras (energy centers in the body), and seated meditation practices. Yoga is for mind, body, *and* spirit and can be a true spiritual practice of devotion, celebration, and joy no matter what your religious beliefs are. Finally we'll put the poses we learned into sequences for desired effects. In sequences we move from one pose to the next without stopping; a constant flow moving with breath and awareness. These sequences are meant to be prescriptive, so whether you're looking for something to energize you in the morning, help you deal with stress, or ease back pain you'll find it here.

In the back of the book, you'll find a glossary of frequently used yoga terms and a list of resources for further learning.

You can start at the beginning of the book and work your way through as knowledge builds and grows. Or you can dip into sections of the book, taking what you need for a certain ailment or curiosity. I hope you find this exploration of yoga easy and informative. Yoga is a deep practice; this book is by no means meant to be inclusive of this depth. It is meant to spark and inspire and give you the beginnings of a positive relationship with yoga. Start where you are! Now is the perfect time to do yoga.

Tools of the Trade

One of the wonderful things about yoga is it does not require any special equipment. To practice yoga all you really need is your breath and your body. In fact, because breathing exercises are so powerful in yoga practice, I always say as long as you can breathe there is some yoga you can do!

That said, there are some great tools that can aid our yoga practice. In this section I'll introduce you to some of the common tools of the trade which can help both in a home practice or in a studio class. Even if you choose not to use these objects it's nice to know how they work.

If you are setting up a home yoga practice, try to set aside a corner of a room just for yoga. This can be a sacred space for your practice. If you do not have a corner free just for yoga, perhaps you can designate a space that can transform into your yoga spot when needed!

Clutter in a space leads to clutter in the mind, so move away anything unnecessary and make sure the floor is clean. Of course, if there is a TV, radio, or computer nearby be sure to turn it off. Put your cell phone away, too! Your yoga corner should be a space that brings you a feeling of calm, a break from external stimuli.

Yoga Mat

One of the most commonly used tools is the yoga mat, which is intended to prevent injury. Typically a long rectangle made of natural jute, rubber, or PVC, the main purpose of a yoga mat is to provide you with a non-slip and cushioned surface. Most mats are around 4 mm thick, enough to provide cushion for feet, hands, and legs. Mats can also be useful in yoga classes for delineating space. Your yoga mat is your little world, a place to breathe deeply, stretch fully, drop stress, and get to know yourself.

Mats roll up easily and many yogis carry their mats in special cylindrical bags made of cloth or nylon. Some people have yoga slings made of just thick straps. Yoga mats are commonly stored rolled up or folded in threes and stacked.

To care for a yoga mat, spray with a natural disinfectant such as Tea Tree Oil between uses, or wipe down with a warm wet cloth and allow the mat to air dry. Some mats can be machine washed, but be sure to check with the manufacturer first!

Some people say our yoga mats absorb the positive energy we put forth in our yoga practice. By caring for and respecting our yoga mats we can show gratitude to both ourselves and the yoga practice!

Yoga Strap

Yoga straps are tools to help you extend your reach. Usually made of cotton or hemp with a metal buckle, a yoga strap can be either hooked into a loop or held straight in a line. Yoga straps are often used by practitioners who cannot touch their toes yet in a shape but hope to feel the sensation another yogi might while touching toes. Sometimes yogis use straps simply because they want to move deeper into a stretch than they'd be able to alone. With breath aiding (inhaling for extension, exhaling to fold deeper into stretches), a yoga strap can help you reach from here to there.

If you do not have a yoga strap handy, you can also use a thin blanket or towel to help you extend your reach. Sometimes yogis even grab hold of their clothing in lieu of using a strap.

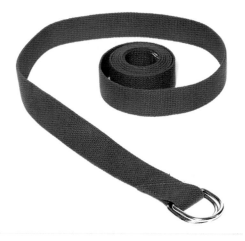

Yoga Block

Yoga blocks are another tool to help us extend our reach in poses and find stability in our shapes. For example, if you are in a standing pose such as Half Moon and hope to touch your fingertips to the floor but can't just yet, a block under your fingers will bring the floor up to you, allowing you to maintain alignment. Sometimes yoga blocks are used as a prop for support. For example, in Bridge pose you may place a block under the small of your back to allow the pose to be more restorative. With the block there, you can rest in the shape, feeling the effects without the effort of holding the shape without a support.

All yoga poses are about alignment and energy. We want to find an open, stable, expansive alignment in all shapes to let energy move through the body freely and most effectively. This prop can help us line up right.

Yoga blocks are usually around 9 inches wide, 6 inches high, and 4 inches deep in measurement. Most are made of foam or cork; something both stable and soft.

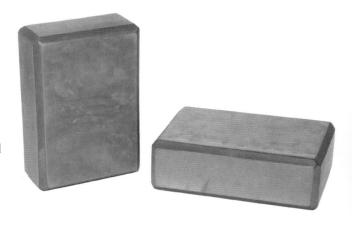

idiot's guides: yoga

Yoga Blanket

Sometimes a folded blanket is just what is needed to help us find stable and easeful alignment in a pose. In many yoga studios you'll find colorful, striped Mexican Blankets. These blankets fold easily into a variety of rectangle sizes and can be used to prop up part of the body in a pose. They can also be comfortably sat upon to lift the hips slightly, encouraging a straight, tall back in a seated posture. Yoga blankets can also be rolled. For example, in Corpse Pose (*Savasana*) you can roll a blanket and place it under your knees to change the alignment and provide a feeling of relief in your lower back.

Yoga blankets can also be used just like, well, blankets! A folded blanket resting on the body in restorative shapes can add extra weight and soft comfort. It can be nice, for example, to place a folded blanket over your hips in Corpse Pose to encourage a sensation of melting into the mat. Sometimes the blankets can also be used for warmth. If you are sitting and practicing your breathing exercises (*pranayama*) or meditation for some time and feel chilly, a yoga blanket wrapped around the body can minimize this distraction and, again, add a feeling of comfort.

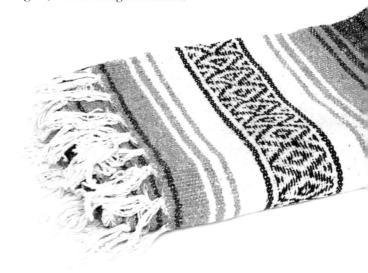

I took a deep breath and listened to the old brag of my heart. I am, I am, I am.

— Sylvia Plath

BREATHING

Breathing (Pranayama)

Breathing is a very important part of yoga practice. *Prana* translates to "life energy" or "life force," symbolized by the breath. *Pranayama* as a whole means an extension of, or drawing out of, life force. By learning how to use your breath, you affect your life energy.

Ancient yogis noticed just how connected our breath is to our emotions and mental states. Think, for example, about how you naturally breathe when you are tired. You might naturally yawn as a call to increase oxygen to the body and wake up! Or you might sigh, letting the air fall out of your mouth and nose. When you are frustrated your breath might become more of a huff and puff. When you are frightened, the breath naturally becomes short and sharp, stuck in the upper chest. The ancient yogis realized that the pattern could also be reversed. By changing the breath, they figured, we could consciously change how we feel. By elongating the breath, they found, we feel calmer. By making the breath short, sharp, and rhythmic, as in Breath of Fire, we feel more energy. Turns out some of our calming, slower breaths can soothe the nervous system and even lower blood pressure and heart rate. Breath is powerful!

Breath is a ticket into the present moment. After all, it is always happening *now*. By paying attention to our inhales and exhales, we bring our minds to the present moment. The breath is a way to check in, be mindful and aware, let worries about the past and future fall away, and note what is actually present and what is just in the mind. This power is always with us.

By learning how to use your breath and paying attention to inhales and exhales, yoga becomes a transformative practice touching mind, body, and spirit all at once. Many say the breath is a bridge between the body, mind, and spirit—yoga means "yoke" or "unify" after all!

As we learn these breathing techniques, please note that breathwork can be done in yoga practice—sometimes during poses or sometimes seated before or after pose work—but it can also be done in any moment of life. To calm down quickly you'll be able to utilize your Three Part Breath, for example, anytime and anywhere. If you get frustrated while out in the world, a quick Lion's Breath will help dispel tension! It's fun to think of creative ways *pranayama* might show up in your life.

In yoga, breath is a type of language. See what your breath is saying to you. Whenever it gets tight or held in pose practice, this may be your body's way of telling you to step back a bit in the shape. In general, inhales are opportunities to extend, stretch, grow large, and exhales are chances to deepen and sink into the moment and pose. Also, inhales are all about welcoming the new and exhales are moments to let go of the past.

Victorious Breath (Ujjayi)

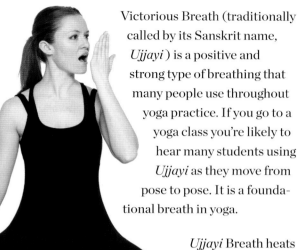

Victorious Breath (traditionally called by its Sanskrit name, *Ujjayi*) is a positive and strong type of breathing that many people use throughout yoga practice. If you go to a yoga class you're likely to hear many students using *Ujjayi* as they move from pose to pose. It is a foundational breath in yoga.

Ujjayi Breath heats the body from the inside out, facilitating our deeper stretches and increased mindfulness. It is also an audible breath that can be used to guide us as we move from pose to pose. For example, if we inhale into one shape, then exhale into another, having a breath we can hear guides us so the breath takes the lead. You may find this breath sounds like the ocean tide, or what you might hear if you hold a conch shell up to your ear. Some people even say it sounds like Darth Vader breathing. However you describe it, it's a wonderful tool for yoga practice.

Ujjayi is done through the nose only, with the lips lightly sealed. We will learn *Ujjayi* first with an open mouth but will gently seal the lips once we've got the technique down.

Step 1: Sit up nice and tall, and place one hand in front of your mouth. Think of this hand as a little mirror, which you are about to fog up using only breath.

Step 2: Take a big breath in, then exhale, fogging up your "mirror." Do this for several rounds to feel and hear this fogging breath.

To practice *Ujjayi* with your mouth closed:

Step 1: Gently close your lips. Take a breath in through your nose.

Step 2: Exhale, making the same fogging sound but this time with your mouth closed. See if you can hear the breath pooling in the back of your throat.

Step 3: Inhale and exhale this way for several rounds, hearing the fogging sound with each exhale.

Step 4: To release this breath practice, on the final exhale allow your lips to open and exhale the air out gently. Return to normal breathing.

Once you learn *Ujjayi* you can take it into your whole yoga practice! In general we inhale when we extend and open the front body in a pose, and we exhale when we forward fold, or release. See if you can move through a pose, feeling inhales as you reach and exhales where you let go. Let the *Ujjayi* Breath guide your exploration.

Three Part Breath

It's a fact that many of us go through our days with shallow breath, utilizing just the lungs and upper chest. With this exercise we go deeper, breathing into the "three:" first the belly, then the chest, and finally the throat. The evenness of inhales and exhales soothe the nervous system and calm the mind. Once you learn it, you can try this breath anytime, anywhere to calm and center yourself. It's relaxation on the go!

Note: Gently seal your lips and breathe in and out of your nose only.

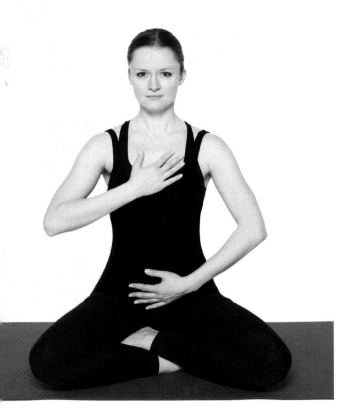

Step 1: Get into a comfortable position, either sitting on the floor with your legs criss-crossed, or lying on your back. Place one hand on your belly and one over your heart.

Step 2: Take a moment to feel your heartbeat. See if you can sense where you have tension in your body and release it.

Step 3: Empty all the air out of your lungs.

Step 4: Begin your inhale from the base of your belly. Feel your belly push out against your hand as you take in air.

Step 5: Continue inhaling into the chest space, to fill your lungs.

Step 6: Continue inhaling into the throat space. Hold the breath for a moment.

Step 7: Exhale slowly, moving in reverse through the throat area, then chest, then belly. Feel your chest and belly collapse as you empty all of the air out of your lungs.

Try this breath between 5 and 10 times. Notice how different you feel after several rounds of Three Part Breath! Noting this difference for yourself will show you how powerful the tool of the breath is.

Alternate Nostril Breath

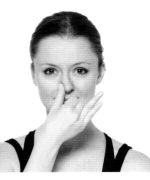

In Alternate Nostril Breath, we use just one nostril at a time to breathe. This is a very even breath, leading to an even state of mind, emotion, and mood. I recently taught this breath to a friend who does not normally practice yoga and she was amazed to feel how, after just a few rounds, she felt very calm and open—as if she'd had a long vacation and drank lots of chamomile tea! All this after only a few breaths. This is the power of *pranayama!*

Step 1: For this *pranayama* you'll need a special hand position (called a *mudra*). Let your left hand rest on your left thigh. Bring your right hand up, curling your pointer and middle finger (your two "peace sign" fingers) into your palm. Leave your thumb, ring finger, and pinky extended, almost in a "hang ten" shape.

Step 2: Start by first taking two to three deep inhales and exhales, utilizing both nostrils.

Step 3: On an exhale, gently push into your right nostril with your thumb, allowing the exhale to flow out of your left nostril only.

Step 4: Inhale through your left nostril.

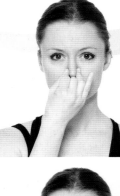

Step 5: Use your ring finger and thumb to momentarily close off both nostrils.

Step 6: Release your thumb and exhale from your right nostril, gently pressing into your left nostril with your ring finger.

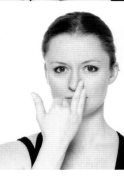

Step 7: Inhale through your right nostril.

Step 8: Repeat, closing off both nostrils and holding, then releasing your fingers and exhaling from the left. Continue this for several rounds.

Step 9: End on your left side with an exhale. After this practice, let your hands fall to your thighs and simply breathe naturally for several breaths. Notice if you feel any different after this *pranayama.*

Note: You may notice one nostril is more clogged than the other. That's perfectly natural! In fact, you may find if you practice this in the morning and then again at night, during the course of one day the openness of your nostrils change. Simply breathe the best you can and don't worry if one nostril flows more than the other.

Breath of Fire

Breath of Fire is a rapid, energizing breath that stimulates the body, giving you a natural energy boost. This breathing exercise will also clear any mental cobwebs, helping you to focus. It is said this breath fires up metabolism, heating up digestive power. It can also lift depression and cut through jangled nerves to help you find an elevated sense of calm.

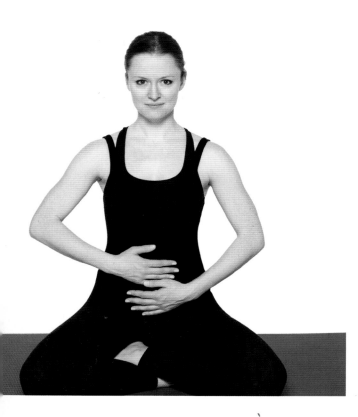

Step 1: Sit up tall. Take a few normal breaths.

Step 2: Take three breaths, focusing on the exhale. Let the breaths be full and complete, cleansing out all air with each exhale.

Step 3: Begin short, sharp, even inhales and exhales through your mouth, pulling your navel in to your spine on the exhales. (In other exercises we push the belly out with an exhale, but here that is reversed! Use a gentle hand placed on your belly to make sure you're moving in the right direction.)

Step 4: Take three more breaths, focusing on the exhale again, making the exhale a bit longer than the inhale.

Step 5: Try this breath for up to 3 minutes to start! You can always work your way up to longer.

Sometimes in practicing Breath of Fire there's a moment where you may feel short of breath from changing the breathing pattern so much. See if you can keep going. If you move through this feeling, it will shift and change.

Take the time to notice, as always, how you feel after Breath of Fire. While many people find it energizing, some find it makes them feel a little nervous or anxious!

Lion's Breath

Lion's Breath is a cleansing breath and is a great way to exhale your stress! Because there is a strong focus on the exhalation, it's also a way to practice letting go. Try this breath both seated and in a pose.

Step 1: Sit up tall with a straight back and open heart. Let your hands rest on your knees, palms up. Take a few normal breaths.

Step 2: Close your mouth and inhale through your nose.

Step 3: Open your mouth, stick out your tongue, and exhale. Sometimes it's fun to scrunch your face, too—allow yourself to expel any frustration or excess energy!

Step 4: After a full exhale, close your mouth and inhale through your nose.

Step 5: Repeat for five breaths, or as many as feels right.

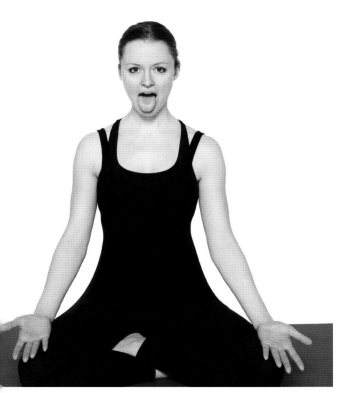

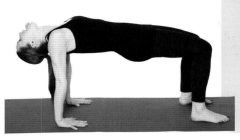

This breath sometimes shows up in yoga classes in different poses. Tabletop Pose is often used for practicing Lion's Breath. With the head back and openness in the throat and front body, this pose is a great place to practice further letting go with the Lion's Breath.

PART

2

THE POSES

Breathing in, I calm body and mind. Breathing out, I smile. Dwelling in the present moment I know this is the only moment.

-Thich Nhat Hanh

GROUNDING

The poses in this section help to bring us down to earth, literally and metaphorically. Many of these postures are on the ground, close to it, or help strengthen and cultivate awareness in the lower body. Because the focus is on bringing the energy downward and finding a steady, stable seat in these postures, stress and the swirling worries of the mind can be calmed.

Keep in mind that all poses touch on many qualities. You'll find that as you ground the body, mind, and energy in these shapes, you're often practicing flexibility, strength, or balance as well. Yoga is wonderfully inclusive in this way.

Keep this section of the book handy for days when you feel too "in your head" or carried away by stress. Taking a few moments to practice a grounding pose can remind us that the earth is under us and we are well, cared for, and safe and sound in this moment—the present moment, breath by breath.

Seated Wide Leg Straddle

Seated Wide Leg Straddle (*Upavistha Konasana*) is sometimes also called a Wide-Angle Seated Forward Bend. This pose provides a deep stretch in the inner thighs, hips, groin, and spine while calming the mind. If you have a lower back injury, be gentle.

SKILL LEVEL
●○○○○

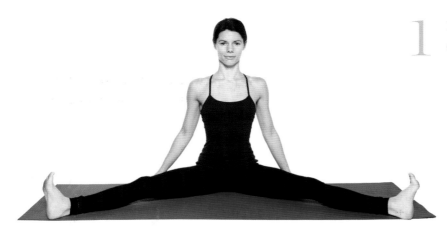

1 Begin sitting up tall, legs stretched out to either side, feet flexed.

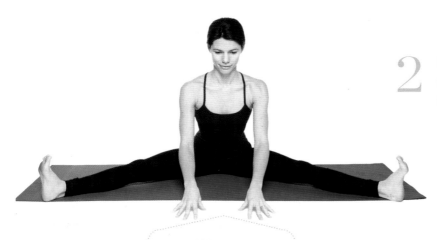

2 Inhale, then exhale and walk your fingers forward. Bend forward at the waist.

Think of extending out and forward from the heart.

If you have a lower back injury or simply need a lift to feel more comfortable in this shape, try placing a folded blanket under your hips.

Stay for 5 to 8 breaths. With each exhale imagine sinking lower toward the floor.

3 Come forward until your elbows are on the floor, fingers splayed wide.

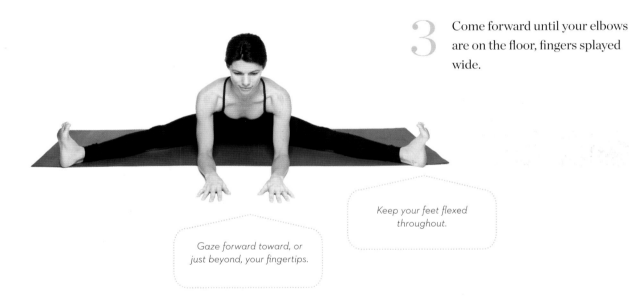

Keep your feet flexed throughout.

Gaze forward toward, or just beyond, your fingertips.

release On an exhale, begin to walk your fingertips back toward your seat. Come to sit up tall, then slowly bring your legs together to touch. Sometimes it's nice to shake out your legs a bit, releasing any tension.

Low Squat

Low Squat (*Malasana*) is also known as Garland Pose. It's a deep, grounding squat that stretches the lower back, groin, and ankles. Proceed with caution if you have knee or lower back sensitivity.

SKILL LEVEL
● ○ ○ ○ ○

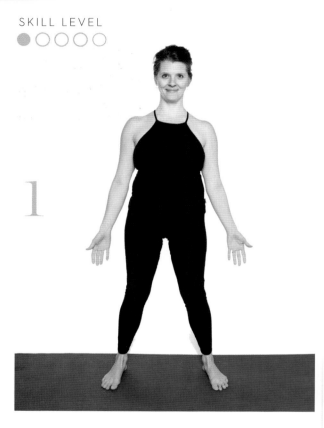

1

Begin in Mountain Pose with your arms at your sides and legs shoulder-width apart.

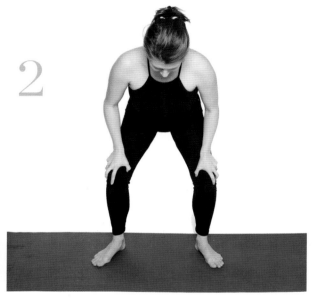

2

Place your hands right above your knees and slowly lower yourself into a squat.

If your heels don't reach, fold a mat or blanket under them for support.

For additional support, stack two blocks and lower yourself down onto them. Aim to keep your back straight, heart gently lifting.

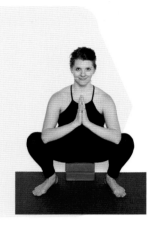

Gaze straight ahead.

3

Aim for your heels to rest on the mat.

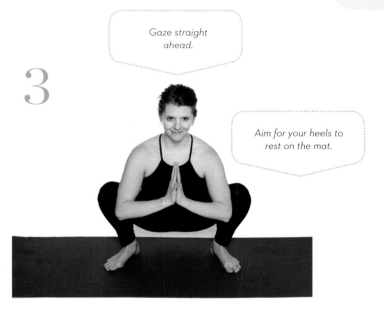

Allow your upper arms to rest against the inside of your thighs. Bring your hands to prayer position.

release   To release Low Squat, drop your hands from the prayer position, bring your hands to the earth or your knees, and start to slowly roll up to standing.

Staff

Staff Pose (*Dandasana*) looks simple, but there's more to this shape than meets the eye! This pose strengthens the arms, shoulders, chest, and back while improving posture. Avoid or proceed carefully if you have a wrist injury.

SKILL LEVEL
● ○ ○ ○ ○

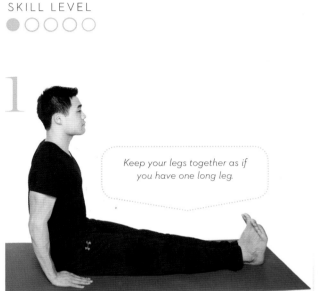

1

Keep your legs together as if you have one long leg.

Begin in a seated position, legs extended straight out. Flex your feet. Place your hands by your hips.

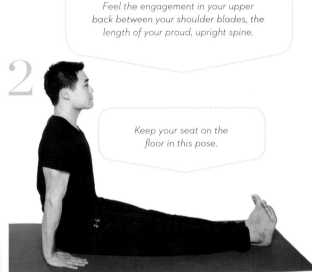

2

Feel the engagement in your upper back between your shoulder blades, the length of your proud, upright spine.

Keep your seat on the floor in this pose.

Press into the earth with your arms so they straighten, and the heart is lifted. Stay for several breath cycles.

keep it easy

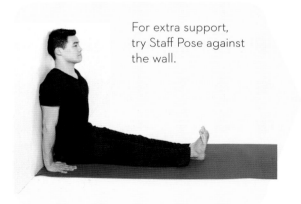

For extra support, try Staff Pose against the wall.

Hero's Pose

Hero's Pose (*Virasana*) is a common seated posture in yoga practice. Here we sit with tall backs and open hearts like the heroes we are. The folded leg position stretches thighs, knees, and ankles. This pose can help reduce leg swelling in the first two trimesters of pregnancy. Avoid if you have any knee injuries or pain.

SKILL LEVEL
● ○ ○ ○ ○

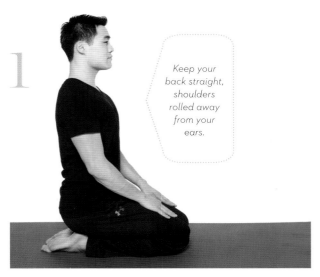

1

Keep your back straight, shoulders rolled away from your ears.

Begin by sitting on your heels with your legs folded under you so the tops of your feet rest on the mat. Rest your palms on your thighs.

keep it easy

If you have less flexibility in your legs or feel any strain through the knees, try sitting on a blanket to raise your hips. Often this lifted seat helps keep the heart lifted and back straight.

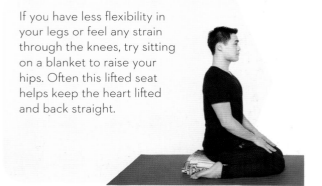

variation

Keeping your knees together, allow your feet to part so there is space for your seat to fall closer to the mat. See if your seat can touch the mat completely while the tops of your feet touch the mat on the outsides of your hips. Keep palms face down in a grounding and calming gesture.

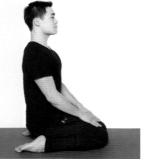

Butterfly

Butterfly Pose (*Badhakonasana*) is sometimes also called Cobbler's Pose, because this is the traditional way cobblers in India sit while working. Here, the legs take the shape of butterfly wings. Butterfly Pose provides a great stretch for the inside of the legs and the groin.

SKILL LEVEL
● ● ○ ○ ○

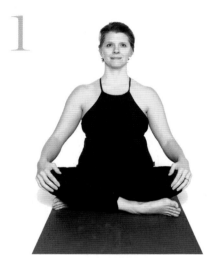

Start in Easy Seat, straight back, hands resting on your knees.

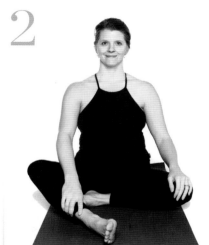

Bring your right foot out in front of you, lining the right sole up with the middle of your body.

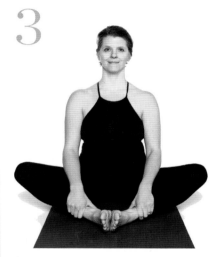

Bring your left foot out and put the soles of your feet together.

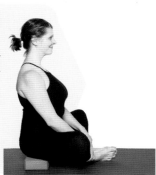

Sit on a block to raise your hips and don't bring your feet in as far to your seat. Keep your Butterfly easy.

Keep your back straight.

Gaze downward a few inches in front of your toes to maintain length in your spine.

Let the heart lead. Think of extending out, then down.

4

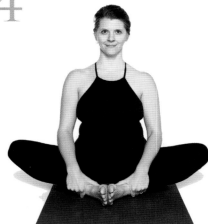

With your hands on your ankles, pull your heels in toward your seat. Sit up tall.

5

Place your hands on the outside of your feet and open up soles of your feet with your thumbs. Let your knees fall open.

6

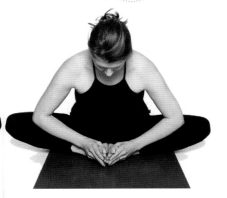

Close your soles and place your elbows on your shins. Exhale, leaning forward. Let your head drop.

release   Slowly come to sit upright, then transition into Easy Seat once again. Feel free to also stretch your legs out straight and give them a shake to loosen them.

Diamond

Diamond Pose (*Tarasana*) is also known as Star Pose. In this posture we bring the legs into a diamond shape. When the torso folds forward, we make the shape of a star. This pose offers a relaxed groin and inner thigh and back body stretch.

SKILL LEVEL

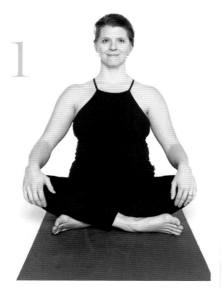

Start in Easy Seat with a straight back, hands resting on your knees.

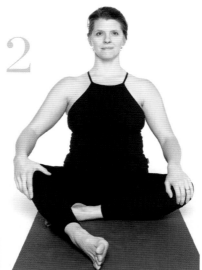

Bring your right foot out in front of you.

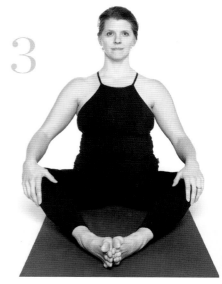

Bring your left foot out, putting the soles of your feet together. Let your knees fall open, making a diamond shape with your legs.

This shape is similar to Butterfly Pose but here the feet rest further out from the seat than in Butterfly. See if you can bring your forehead to your feet. If not, simply relax forward without strain or pulling. Either gaze at your feet or let your head drop.

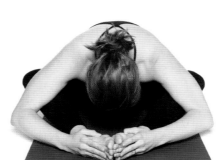

If your hips are tight, place blocks under your knees for support.

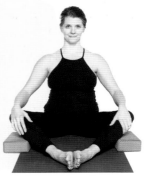

4

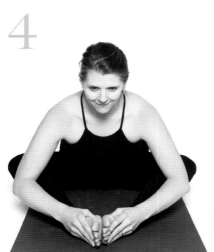

Place your hands on your feet, thumbs on your instep. Exhale and fold forward, with knees staying wide.

5

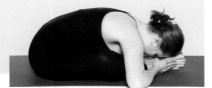

Relax your neck and let your head drop.

release   To release, sit upright. Either bring your feet toward your seat and resume Easy Seat, or or just straighten your legs.

Seated One-Leg Forward Fold

Seated One Leg Forward Fold (*Janu Sirsasana*) is also known as Head-to-Knee Forward Bend. Here we are folding forward so the head reaches toward the knee. This pose calms the mind; stretches the hamstrings, groin, and spine; and helps relieve anxiety and fatigue.

SKILL LEVEL
●●○○○

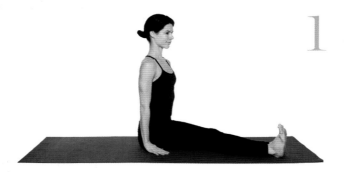

1 Begin in Staff Pose, legs straight on the floor, toes pointed up.

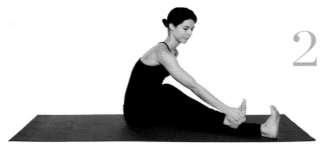

2 Reach down and grab your right foot. Use your stomach muscles to roll up to sit, bringing your foot along.

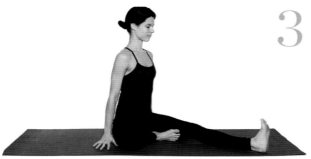

3 Place the sole of your right foot on the inside of your left thigh. Tent your fingers by your hips. Center your torso over the extended left leg.

4

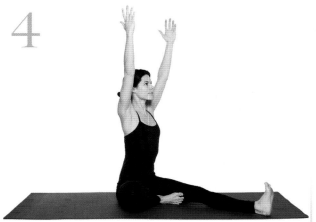

On the inhale, raise your arms over your head, palms facing each other.

5

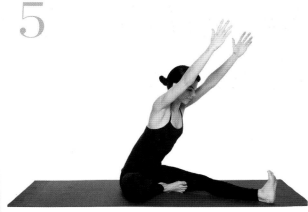

Exhale and bend at the waist, back straight. Lead with the heart, reaching out then down.

6

Keep your back flat.

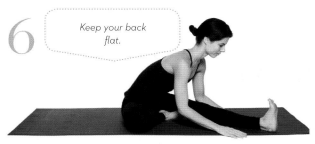

Place your hands on either side of your left leg. Gaze down toward your shin.

7

Don't forget to breathe!

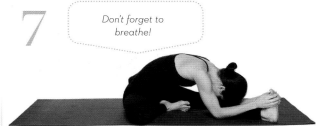

After reaching forward as far as you can, just release, letting your head drop, melting down.

variation

If you're flexible enough, try bringing your foot to the top of your thigh in a half Lotus position. From here you can fold forward with your foot tucked in a Lotus shape.

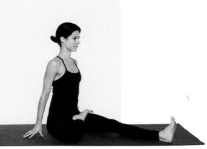

keep it easy

If you have any knee pain or an injury, keep your left knee bent a little. You can also try putting a folded blanket under your right knee.

release   To release, simply walk backward through the steps, landing in Staff Pose. From there, do the other leg!

Seated Two-Leg Forward Fold

Seated Two Leg Forward Fold (*Paschimottanasana*) is also known as Seated Forward Bend. This simple forward fold is powerful: it calms the mind and relieves the blues and stress. It stretches the hamstrings and spine and even improves digestion. If you have any back injury, be gentle or skip this posture.

SKILL LEVEL
● ● ○ ○ ○

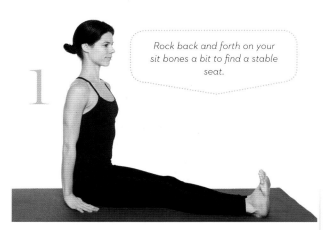

1

Rock back and forth on your sit bones a bit to find a stable seat.

Begin in Staff Pose, legs together, feet flexed.

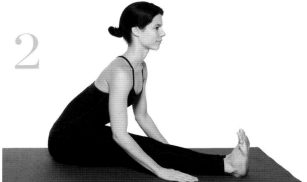

2

Inhale, then exhale, beginning to reach forward through the heart, then down.

Think of extending your heart out and then down in this shape. With each breath, see if you can notice the micro-movements within the shape: the way the heart reaches outward with the inhale and the hips sink deeper with each exhale. Even when we hold a pose there's a lot happening inside!

Gently give into gravity and drop your head.

3

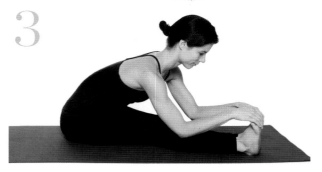

Reach for your toes, feet, or anywhere on your legs. Stay for several breaths, letting gravity deepen the stretch naturally.

keep it easy

There's no need to pull or be forceful in this pose. If you can't reach your feet, ankles, or shins, simply fall forward where you are.

release   On an exhale, simply roll up to sit in Staff Pose once again.

Reclining Hero

We can recline our Hero's Pose (*Virasana*) to achieve a deeper stretch in the front of the legs and hips as well as the abdomen, chest, and throat. Move slowly, noticing sensations as you go. Avoid if you have any knee injury or pain.

SKILL LEVEL
●●●○○

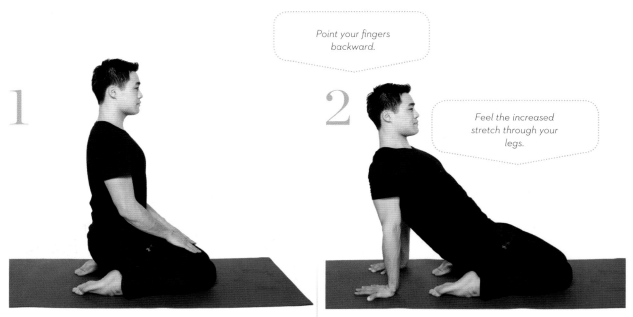

Point your fingers backward.

Feel the increased stretch through your legs.

1

Begin in Hero's Pose variation with knees together but feet apart so the seat reaches the floor, hands on your thighs.

2

Lean back, placing your hands on the mat directly behind your hips. If you are a beginner, you can stop here.

It's normal to feel a bit dizzy or lightheaded after such a large throat and heart opener. Allow yourself to sit upright in Hero's Pose for a few moments after Reclining Hero.

3

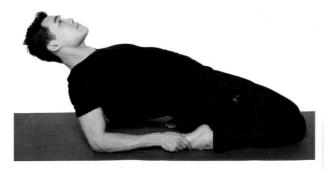

Come down onto your elbows so your forearms rest on the mat. Try to grab your feet with your hands.

4

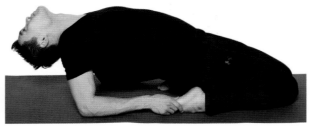

Allow your head to fall back, opening up the throat.

release   Release out of this pose slowly, rewinding through the steps. Find Hero's Pose again, then slowly unwind your legs, coming to sit directly on the mat.

Bend and be straight.

-Tao Te Ching

FLEXIBILITY

When many people think yoga they think "flexibility." It's true that this is a quality many yoga poses help to cultivate. However, it's important to know that there's no need to be super flexible before you hop onto the yoga mat. The only prerequisite to practicing yoga is having the willingness. And if you're holding this book you most likely have that.

That said, the poses in this section are a great place to start if being flexible is high on your list of personal goals. Here we will guide the body into shapes, using breath and intention, to practice flexibility in a variety of body parts. And, in the spirit of the mind-body connection, a flexible body leads to a flexible mind. As you stretch with care and deep breathing, you'll also calm the mind and gently elevate the spirit.

A bonus? Mindfully cultivating balance in the muscles, joints, and connective tissues of the body can help decrease our chances of injury in sports and in life, and can keep us looking and feeling young. As you work on flexibility, you're also working on staying mobile for as long as possible—so breathe deep and stretch well.

Note: Use your deep breathing—your Ujjayi Breath is recommended—to guide the body into deeper stretches. Let the tools of breath and muscle warmth aid you in growing flexible.

Easy Seat

Easy Seat (*Sukhasana*) is just that: a seat that is meant to feel full of ease and comfort while being upright. This shape calms the mind while strengthening the back and core of the body. You will feel firmly connected to the earth with your lower body as you extend upward to the sky with your upper body. Though simple, this is a powerful shape, full of dignity and wisdom. Avoid if you have a serious knee injury.

SKILL LEVEL
● ○ ○ ○ ○

Make your chin parallel with the mat.

It is normal for your feet to fall asleep in this pose, especially when you're getting used to the shape. You can shift your leg position, as long as you maintain your calm, stable state of mind.

Feel the strength of the back of your body supporting you.

Feel your lungs open up.

An upright and aligned position allows for energy to flow freely.

1

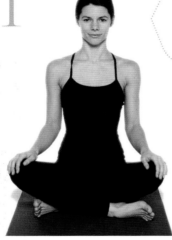

Sit with your legs crossed, hands resting on your thighs. Roll your shoulders back and down, creating an opening in the heart space. Exhale and let go of any tension you feel throughout your body.

keep it easy

Sit on a blanket to raise your hips above your knees.

If you have knee pain, try sitting in a looser pretzel shape.

If you have a lot of back pain, it is ok to sit along a wall. Just be sure you are still finding alignment and engaging the core lightly. Don't just lean on the wall!

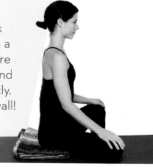

Standing Side Stretch

Standing Side Stretch (*Parsva Tadasana*) provides a wonderful feeling of length along the side of the body from hips to fingertips. Here, you get to stretch areas that aren't often reached. This move improves posture and contributes to spine health.

SKILL LEVEL
● ○ ○ ○ ○

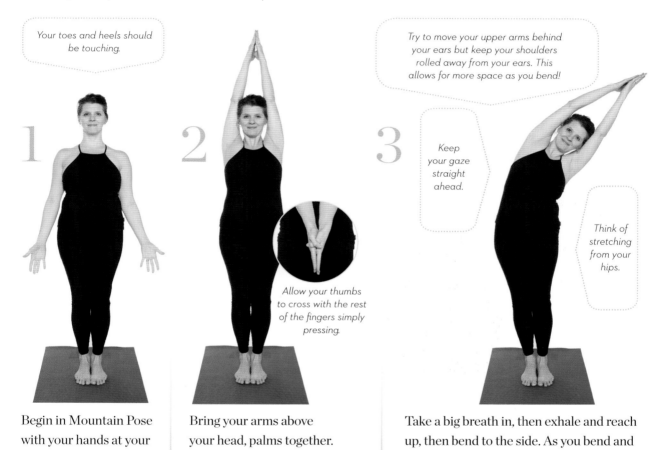

Your toes and heels should be touching.

Try to move your upper arms behind your ears but keep your shoulders rolled away from your ears. This allows for more space as you bend!

Keep your gaze straight ahead.

Allow your thumbs to cross with the rest of the fingers simply pressing.

Think of stretching from your hips.

1
Begin in Mountain Pose with your hands at your sides, feet together.

2
Bring your arms above your head, palms together.

3
Take a big breath in, then exhale and reach up, then bend to the side. As you bend and stretch, press your palms together.

release To release, inhale then exhale, returning to an upright standing position. Don't forget to then bend to the other side.

Wrist Flexion

It is important to stretch the wrists and ankles to maintain a healthy range of motion. While doing these exercises, remind yourself of all the work your hands and feet do for you daily, and send some gratitude toward those parts of the body.

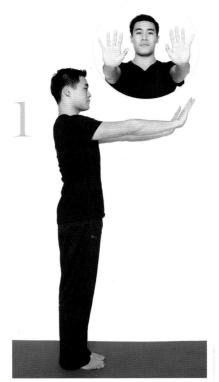

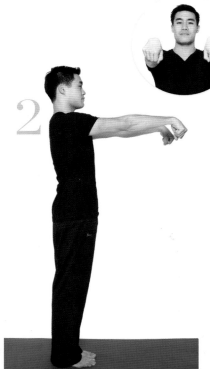

Wrist Flexion can be especially helpful if you've been typing or working at a desk for many hours.

Start with your arms up, hands in line with your shoulders. Spread your fingers wide and gaze ahead.

Drop your hands down, feeling the pull in the top of your hand and wrist. Gently curl your fingers in to your palms.

Foot Flexion

1

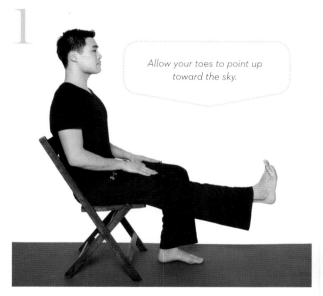

Allow your toes to point up toward the sky.

Sit in a chair, keeping your back straight and shoulders relaxed. Straighten your knee and flex your foot.

2

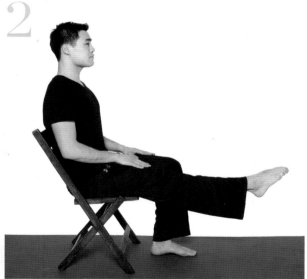

Point your toes. Feel the gentle stretch in your ankle.

Shoulder Roll

Shoulder Rolls help release stress from the upper back, chest, and shoulders themselves. They can be done seated or standing and are a quick way to drop tension. Shoulder Rolls can be helpful after a long day of sitting at a desk typing or after carrying heavy bags and packages, for example.

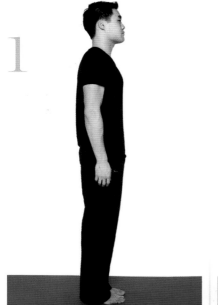

1

Begin in Mountain Pose, arms relaxed at your sides.

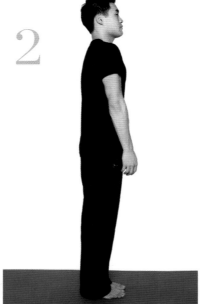

2

Bring your shoulders forward, stretching out your back.

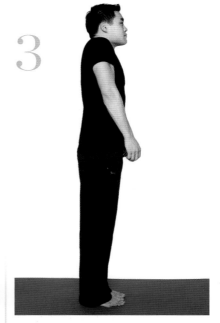

3

Bring your shoulders up to your ears.

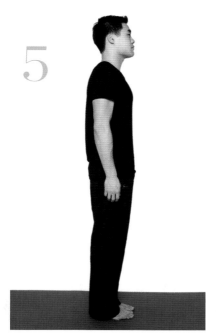

Try reversing directions starting with the backward motion, then moving up, and then forward.

The cycle of movement is connected with the cycle of breath. Exhale as you bring your shoulders forward, inhale as you bring them toward the ears, and exhale as you bring your shoulders back and down.

4

Drop your shoulders back, imagining your shoulder blades could touch.

5

Come back to the original position.

Child's Pose

Child's Pose (*Balasana*) is a restful shape. Often this posture comes at the beginning and end of yoga sequences. Whenever you need a break in yoga, try Child's Pose. This posture stretches the hips, thighs, and back; calms the mind; and relieves stress. If your back is sensitive, try one of the "Keep It Easy" variations.

SKILL LEVEL

● ○ ○ ○ ○

It's nice to stay in this shape for several breaths or even several minutes. Really allow yourself to relax.

1

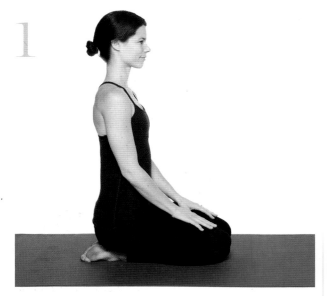

Begin in Hero's Pose with your hips resting on your heels and your hands resting on your thighs .

2

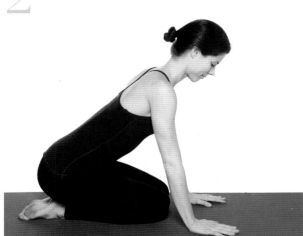

Shift your weight forward and place your hands on the mat.

Let your knees spread out wide
so your torso can relax in between them. Extend your arms,
palms face down. Feel the extra
space created. Breathe!

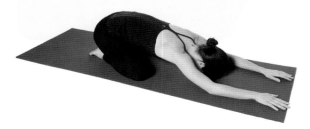

For a little extra support in your
Child's Pose, place a folded
blanket between your shins and
thighs.

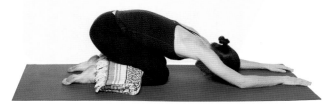

3

*Allow the mat to fully support
you as you release all muscle
and mental tension.*

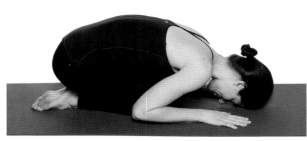

Bring your forehead to rest on the mat. Your torso
can rest gently on your thighs with your back relaxed.
There's no sensation of holding here. Your whole job is
to rest.

4

*With each inhale feel the back of
the body expand up and out. With
each exhale, imagine you melt
further into the mat.*

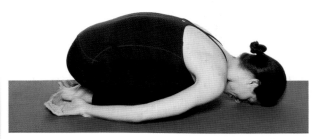

With your forehead on the mat, bring your arms behind you, palms face up. Here we are bowing our heads
to the earth.

release   To release, simply roll up to sit on your heels.

Cat

Cat Pose (*Marjariasana*), provides a wonderful and safe way to stretch the spine and gently massage the organs of the belly. Cat Pose often works hand-in-hand with Cow Pose. Move with breath, performing Cat Pose on an exhale and coming into a neutral all-fours position or Cow Pose with an inhale. If you have a neck injury, keep your head in line with your torso rather than dropping it.

SKILL LEVEL
● ○ ○ ○ ○

1

Keep your elbows straight. Think of rotating the inside of your elbows toward the front of your mat.

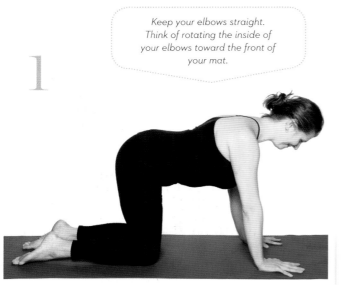

Begin on all fours, aligning your wrists under your shoulders and your knees under your hips. Spread your fingers wide and keep your gaze downward.

2

Allow your head to drop to prevent neck strain. You can shake it "yes" and "no" to release tension.

Gaze toward your belly button. This will allow your neck to drop.

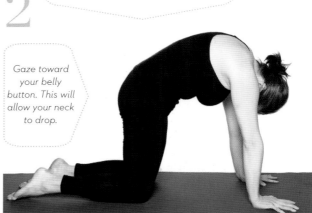

Arch your back, pulling the belly toward the spine. Pull your belly in and up. Imagine your belly-button can touch your backbone.

release To release, simply transition back to all fours on an inhale. From here, you can rest in Child's Pose if desired.

Cow Pose (*Bitilasana*) provides a wonderful way to warm up the spine and stretch the front body. Cow Pose is often paired with Cat Pose. If you have a neck injury, aim to look straight ahead rather than up.

Cow

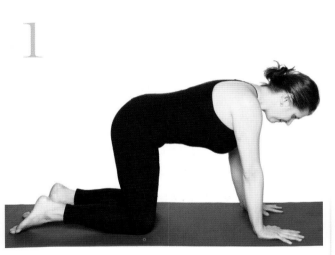

1

Begin on all fours with your wrists under your shoulders and your knees under your hips, and gaze straight down. Spread your fingers wide.

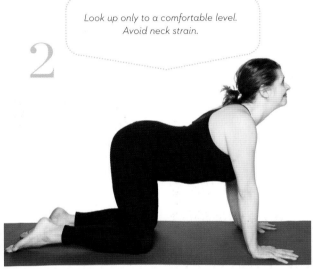

2

Look up only to a comfortable level. Avoid neck strain.

Allow the belly to drop and the heart to expand. Gaze upward, with a sway in your back like a cow's.

release To release, simply transition back to an all fours position. You may then find your Child's Pose to rest.

Seated Spinal Twist

Seated Spinal Twist (*Ardha Matsyendrasana*), sometimes also called Half Lord of the Fishes Pose, twists the spine from a seated position. Here we energize the spine by rotating it, and stimulate digestive organs by "wringing them out." Be sure to twist on both sides! If you are pregnant or dealing with a back injury, try the second variation.

SKILL LEVEL
●●○○○

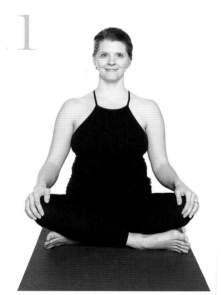

1

Start in Easy Seat with a straight back and hands resting on your knees.

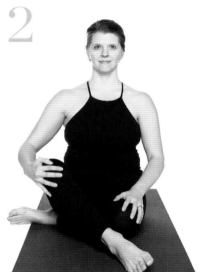

2

Unwind your legs a bit, bringing your left knee to the center of the body.

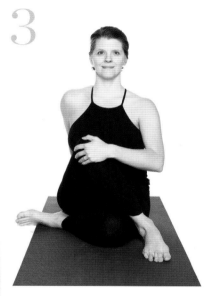

3

Pick up your right foot and place it on the outside of your left knee, sole to the mat.

keep it easy

Variation 1: For a softer variation, keep legs in an Easy Seat position. Bring your left hand to your right knee and gaze forward or gently back over your right shoulder.

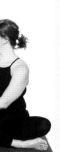

Variation 2: For an even gentler twist, keep your Easy Seat legs, place your right hand on your right knee and tent your left fingertips behind you. Twist softly left.

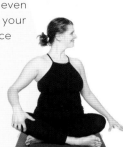

Variation 3: For an extra lift to aid you in keeping the heart upright, consider sitting on a block.

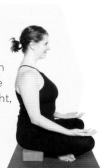

Keep the fingertips of your right hand pressing gently into the mat.

4

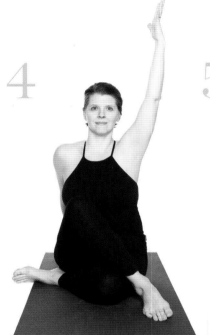

Reach your left arm up to the sky on an inhale.

5

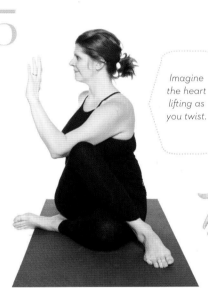

Imagine the heart lifting as you twist.

Exhale, and twist from the bottom of your spine to bring your left arm to the outside of your knee.

6

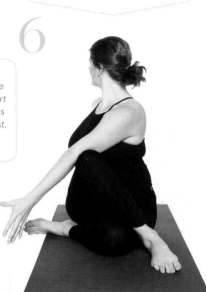

Straighten out your left arm, gently pressing it into the outside of your knee. Look over your right shoulder.

release To release the pose, gently move backward through the above steps. Unwind and find Easy Seat.

Lotus

Lotus Pose (*Padmasana*) is a classic yoga position. In this shape, our hips are elevated slightly to allow for lift in the heart, a straight and open posture. Practicing Lotus regularly is said to help pregnant yogis in childbirth, as there is a strong opening in the hips and lower body. ***Please note:*** not everyone can sit this way simply due to the placement and build of their bone structure! Give Lotus a try, but never force yourself into anything painful.

SKILL LEVEL

●●●○○○

See if you can let both knees melt toward the floor.

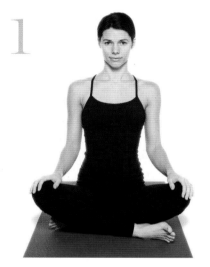

1

Begin in Easy Seat, with your hands resting on your thighs or knees.

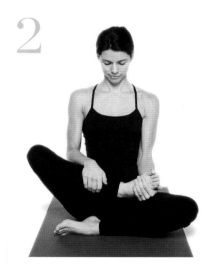

2

Reach for your right foot and leg.

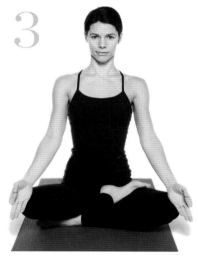

3

Place the top of your right foot on the upper part of your left thigh. Sit up straight, feeling how this position tips your pelvis.

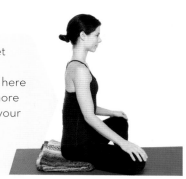

keep it easy

Try placing a blanket under your hips to elevate them. From here you may discover more room to move into your Lotus Pose.

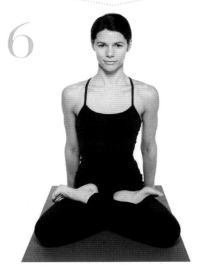

Think of sitting tall and allow your knees to melt toward the mat.

Gaze straight ahead, or close your eyes.

4

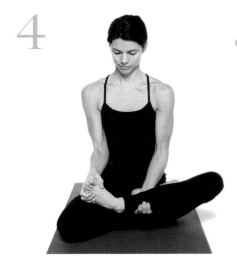

Reach down for your left foot.

5

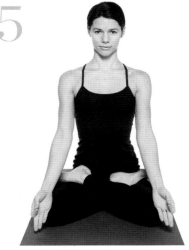

Carefully place your left foot on top of your right thigh. Bring your hands to rest on your knees or allow your index fingers to connect with your thumbs (chin mudra).

6

Flex through your feet. Allow the soles to face the ceiling.

release   To release the pose, simply unwind the steps above, coming to sit in Easy Seat.

Fire Log

Fire Log (*Agnistambhasana*) is often also called "Ankle to Knee" Pose. Indeed here we sit with our ankles and knees stacked, creating the shape of stacked logs. Fire Log provides a wonderful hip stretch.

SKILL LEVEL
●●○○○

> Gaze straight ahead, keeping your chin parallel to the mat.

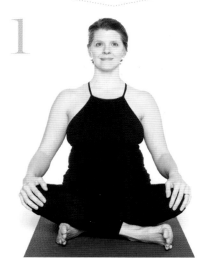

1

Start in Easy Seat with your back straight, hands resting on your knees.

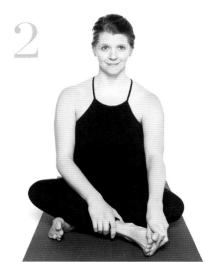

2

Bring your left shin parallel to the front of the mat. Prepare to lift your right foot. Flex through the foot.

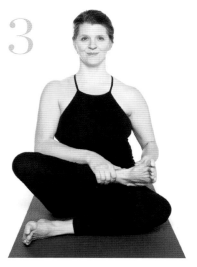

3

Raise your right foot toward your left knee.

For an extra lift
to aid you in
keeping the
heart upright,
consider
sitting on a
block.

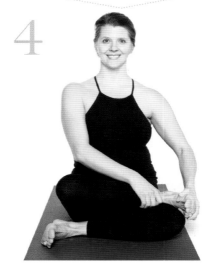

Be sure to rest your ankle on top
of your knee and not your foot to
prevent ankle strain.

keep it easy

If the top knee doesn't
reach the bottom
ankle, feel free to place
a yoga block or folded
blanket between the
knee and ankle for
support.

4

5

Place your right shin on top of
your left leg, lining your ankle up
on your knee.

Flex through both feet. Place your
hands palms down on your thighs
or bring your index fingers and
thumbs to touch (chin mudra).
Maintain a straight back and feel
the stretch through the hips and
lift in the heart.

release   To release, unstack your legs and come into Easy Seat.

Cow Face

Cow Face Pose (*Gomukhasana*) stretches many things at once: ankles, thighs, hips, shoulders, triceps, and the chest. In this shape, with the knees placed one on top of the other, we create the shape of a "cow's head." The extended feet create the shape of horns or floppy ears. Be sure to use one of the arm variations if you have shoulder or neck problems.

SKILL LEVEL
●●○○○

Your heel should be aligned with your hip.

Make sure your ankles are parallel with each other

1

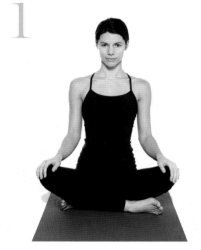

Begin in Easy Seat, hands on knees.

2

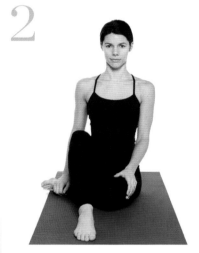

Bring your right foot out in front of you. Move your left knee to the center of your body.

3

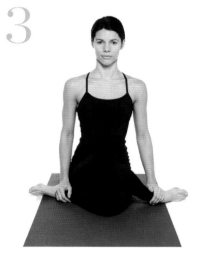

Lift your right leg at the ankle. Place your right foot on the outside of your hip. Stack your knees one on top of the other. Flex your feet.

It's perfectly fine just to find the leg position first, keeping your arms by your side. With just the lower body in Cow Face Pose you'll still find quite a hip and leg stretch! It's also possible to practice the arm position on its own, keeping the legs neutral in a criss-cross position or even standing.

Instead of grasping fingers, hold onto your shirt, or ...

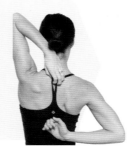

... use a strap

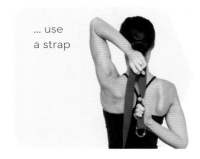

Keep your back straight.

4

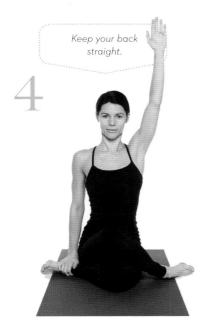

Inhale, extending your left arm up to the sky.

5

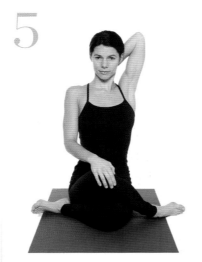

Exhale, bending your left arm at the elbow, placing your left hand on your back between your shoulder blades.

6

See if you can hold hands with yourself behind your back.

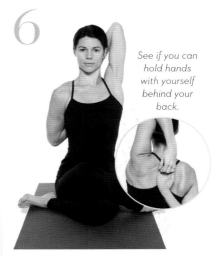

Bring your right behind your back and grasp the fingertips of both hands.

release To release, unwind your arms first, then your legs, coming into Easy Seat.

Thread the Needle

Thread the Needle got its name from its shape: here one arm forms the "eye of the needle" and the other arm forms the thread, weaving through. Thread the Needle is a wonderful shoulder opener and also serves to wring out and twist the spine.

SKILL LEVEL
●●○○○

1

Keep your core engaged and back straight, looking down.

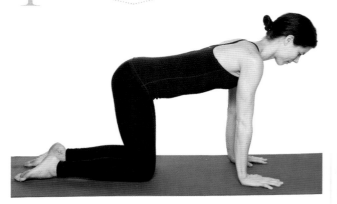

2

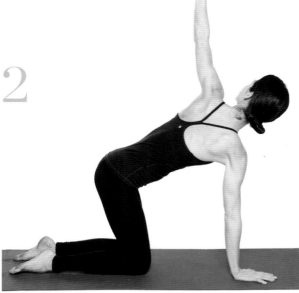

Begin on your hands and knees in an all-fours position. Place your hands under your shoulders, fingers spread wide.

Inhale and reach your left arm up to the ceiling, looking up at your extended fingers.

variation

For a more restorative shape, try Thread the Needle from Child's Pose, with your hips on your heels. If there is any strain in your neck, go back to the elevated version, with hips raised.

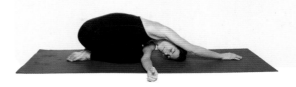

3

Aim to keep your hips square.

Gaze toward your left fingers, or close your eyes.

Your left shoulder should be on the mat.

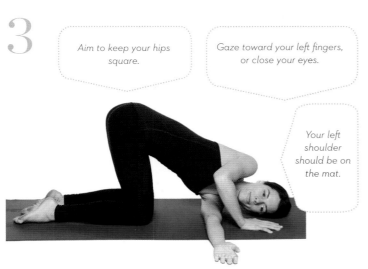

Exhale, and bring your left arm down and through, underneath your right arm. Bring your left ear to the mat.

release

To release, simply draw your left arm back and find your all fours position. From there, move to the other side.

Cobra

Cobra Pose (*Bhujangasana*) is a backbend that strengthens the spine while stretching the abdomen, shoulders, and chest. Cobra stimulates the digestive organs as well. Move mindfully if you have a lower back injury. This pose is not for pregnant yogis.

SKILL LEVEL
● ● ○ ○ ○

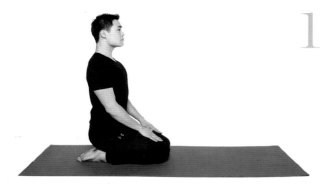

1 Begin in Hero's Pose with your hips resting on your heels and your hands resting on your thighs right above the knees.

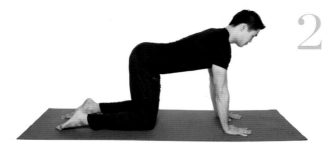

2 Shift your weight forward and place your hands on the mat, coming into an all-fours position. Gaze downward.

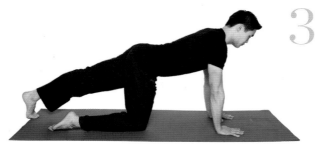

3 Extend your left leg back, curling your toes under. Engage your core so your leg is extending from the center of your body and not simply flung back.

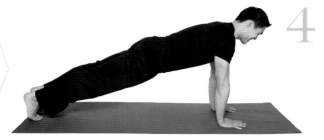

Make sure your wrists are stacked under your shoulders here.

4 Extend your right leg back, also mindfully. Now you are in a Plank position.

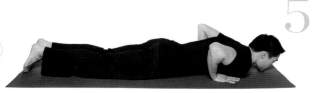

Use your core muscles, your arm muscles, and your patience!

5 Slowly lower yourself down to the mat, coming to lie on your belly. See if you can move slowly and in one solid line.

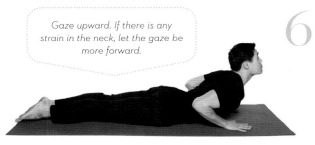

Gaze upward. If there is any strain in the neck, let the gaze be more forward.

6 Place your palms on the mat so your fingertips line up with your shoulders, your elbows bent back and up. Inhale, then exhale and press palms into the floor. Your chest and throat will open up. (This is Baby Cobra; beginners can stop here).

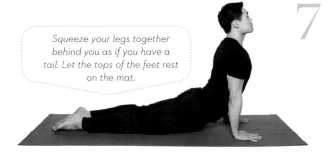

Squeeze your legs together behind you as if you have a tail. Let the tops of the feet rest on the mat.

7 To rise into a bigger Cobra, inhale then exhale and press into the mat with your palms, straightening out your arms. Keep your legs and pelvis on the floor, lifting through the heart.

release Release by moving backward through the steps above. Letting the breath be even and full, slowly lower to your belly. It can be nice to rest on the belly for several breaths, bringing one ear to the mat, before coming up to sit.

Downward Facing Dog

Downward Facing Dog (*Adho Mukha Svanasana*) is one of the most foundational and recognized poses in yoga. It's a pose we naturally transition into as toddlers when we are first learning to walk. The many benefits of this shape include calming the mind and easing mild depression, strengthening the legs and arms, improving digestion and providing energy in the body. Avoid if you are in the last term of pregnancy.

SKILL LEVEL
●●●○○

1

Hands should be shoulder-width apart for a strong base.

Spread your fingers wide and gently press your palms on the mat.

2

Allow for feet to be hip-width apart on the mat. Imagine two fists or your head between your feet to help measure the distance.

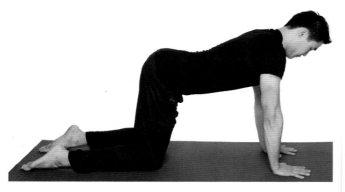

Begin in all-fours position on your hands and knees, back straight. Gaze downward.

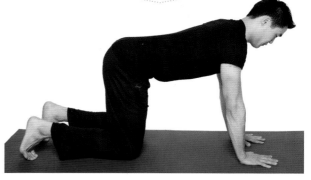

Curl your toes under.

Downward Facing Dog can help prevent osteoporosis and help flat feet. It's a wonderful shape to come into every day, whether you have time for a full practice or not!

Your heels may or may not reach the floor in this shape. What's important is the action of pressing the heels toward the earth. As the back of your legs become more flexible, you will naturally find your heels reaching further toward the floor.

Stay for 3 to 5 deep, full cycles of breath.

3

Keep your fingers spread wide. Feel the energy in all your fingers and your palms as you press gently into the mat.

4

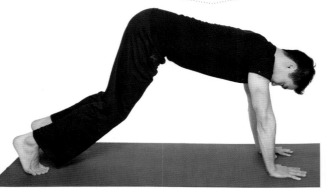

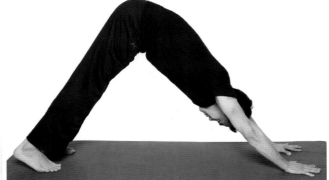

Begin to straighten out your legs, bringing your hips to the sky. Allow your head to drop, no tension in the neck.

Push back into your legs so your hips are high and your heels are low. Again, let your head drop. You can even shake your head and nod it gently to release any stress or holding on.

release   To release, simply bend your knees and transition back to a Child's Pose. It's nice to rest in Child's Pose for several breaths, feeling the effects of Downward Facing Dog on the mind and body.

Upward Facing Dog

Upward Facing Dog (*Urdhva Mukha Svanasana*) strengthens the arms and legs while stretching out the hips, chest, and throat. It is a wonderful backbend, strengthening the spine, also. Upward Facing Dog can improve posture and digestion. Avoid if pregnant; move with caution if you have a back injury.

SKILL LEVEL
● ● ● ○ ○

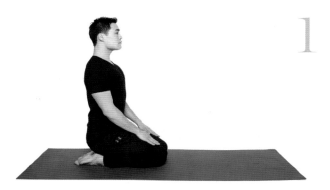

1 Begin in Hero's Pose with your hips resting on your heels and your hands resting on your thighs.

Make sure not to let your back sink. Feel a lift in the heart.

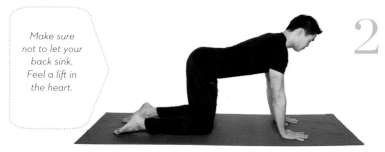

2 Shift your weight forward and place your hands on the mat, coming onto all fours.

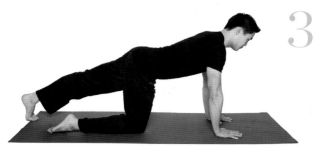

3 Extend your left leg back.

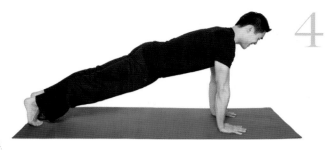

4 Extend your right leg back. (This is Plank Pose.)

Don't let your back bow. If this is difficult, bring your knees to the mat first then lower down.

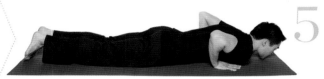

5 Slowly lower yourself down to the mat. Try to lower yourself to the mat in one straight line. Gaze downward.

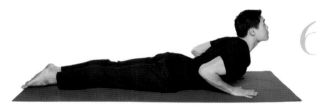

6 Press your palms into the floor and push up your chest.

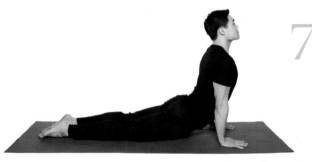

7 Straighten out your arms and lift with your chest.

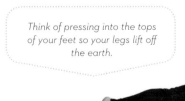

Think of pressing into the tops of your feet so your legs lift off the earth.

8 Press even higher, bringing your hips and thighs off the floor.

Gaze upward. If you feel any neck strain, gaze forward.

release On an exhale, slowly lower your torso to the earth. Come to lie on your belly, letting one ear rest on the mat.

Low Lunge

Low Lunge (*Anjaneyasana*) is sometimes also called Crescent Lunge. This shape provides a deep stretch in the thighs, groin, and chest. It also stretches the psoas muscle, an important muscle deep in the body that helps connect our upper body to the lower and runs along the front of the hip. This pose can help you maintain a healthy back and good posture for life.

SKILL LEVEL
●●●○○

1

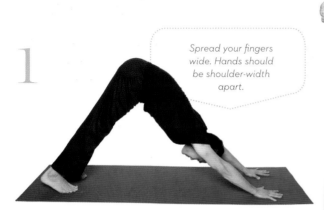

Spread your fingers wide. Hands should be shoulder-width apart.

Begin in Downward Facing Dog, hips high and heels pressing toward the mat.

2

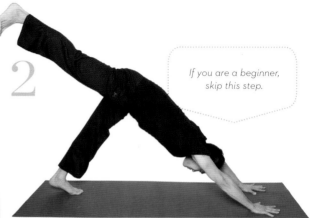

If you are a beginner, skip this step.

Inhale, then exhale, extending your right leg back and up. Keep your hips square. Flex through the raised foot.

3

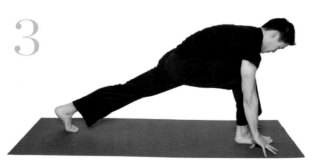

Using your core muscles, step your right foot in between your hands. Place your foot so your toes line up with your fingertips.

4

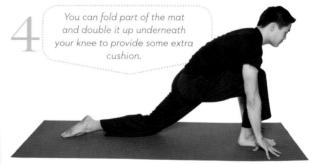

You can fold part of the mat and double it up underneath your knee to provide some extra cushion.

Lower your left knee to the mat. Uncurl the toes of your left foot. Let the top of your foot rest on the mat.

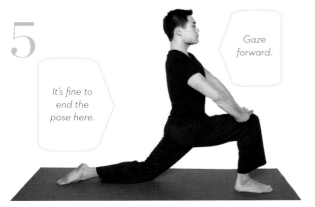

5

It's fine to end the pose here.

Gaze forward.

Bring your hands up and interlace them on top of your right thigh. Gently press your hands into your leg, moving your arms closer to straight, opening the chest.

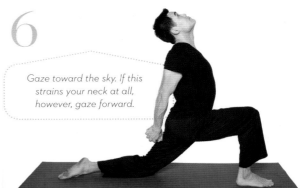

6

Gaze toward the sky. If this strains your neck at all, however, gaze forward.

To aid a feeling of back bend, interlace your fingers behind your back. Inhale, then exhale, straightening out your arms and extending your hands toward the mat.

variation

To further stretch your arms while maintaining a backbend, hook your thumbs together and raise your arms overhead. Gaze toward your fingers.

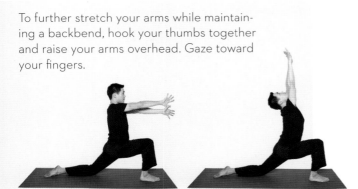

release   To release the shape, bring your hands back to the mat, on either side of the front foot. Slowly step the front foot back so both knees rest on the mat. Press back into Child's Pose.

Lizard

Lizard Pose (*Utthan Pristhasna*) provides a large hip stretch and strengthens the legs and upper body.

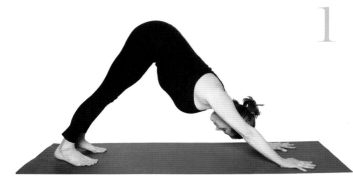

1 Begin in Downward Facing Dog, hips high and heels reaching toward or pressing into the mat.

Your weight should be fairly evenly placed between the front and back body at first. Then begin to feel a bit more weight in your front foot.

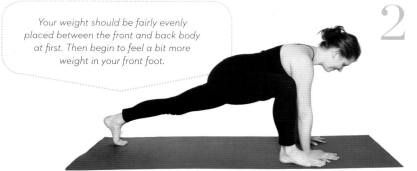

2 Step your right foot forward toward the outside of your right hand. It's ok if it takes a few small steps to arrive.

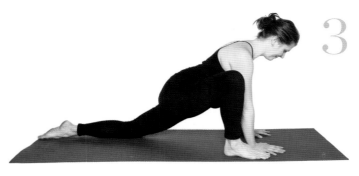

3 Bring your left knee down to the floor, allowing the top of your left foot to rest on the mat. Look downward.

Line up your fingers with your elbows in straight lines. Imagine a straight line of energy from your middle finger through your elbow.

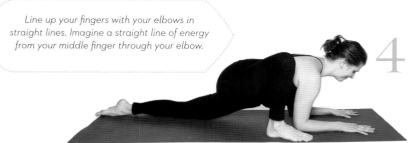

4 Release down onto your elbows with forearms on the mat. Point your fingertips forward.

Gaze downward right in between your wrists, to keep a natural extension in your spine.

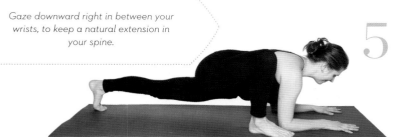

5 For added challenge, tuck your back toes under and lift your back knee up to a straight position. Think of squaring your hips toward the mat.

variation

For more of a stretch in the hip, allow your front foot to roll open to the outside of the foot. Here, your knee and hip can also roll open. Breathe, imagining breath flooding the hip.

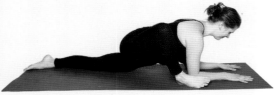

release

To release, allow your left knee to rest on the mat then bring your right knee back to meet it. Press back to Child's Pose.

Rock the Baby

Rock the Baby Pose allows for a stretch through the hip and thigh of the elevated leg. The pose got its name from the way we cradle the shin like a baby.

SKILL LEVEL
●●●○○

Use your left hand and arm to support your leg.

1
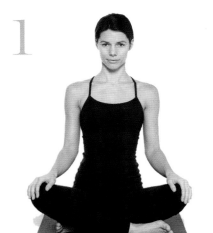

Begin in Easy Seat with legs crossed, palms face down on the legs.

2
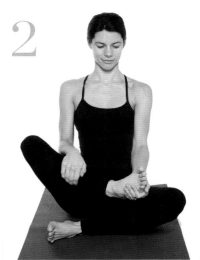

With both hands, grab your right foot and raise it.

3
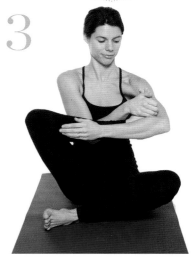

With your right hand, place your foot in the crook of your left elbow.

Feel free to gently rock your shin from side to side, much as you would rock a baby, to engage the stretch.

keep it easy

If you can't bring your foot and knee to the crook of your arms, just hold them with your hands.

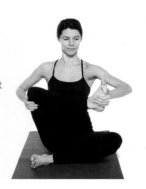

See if you can sit with a straight back and tall heart, even in this shape. Avoid the temptation to slouch.

Gaze straight ahead.

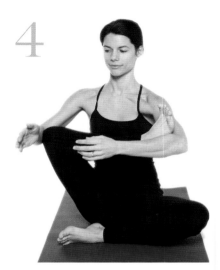

4

Place your right knee in the crook of your right arm. Your shin will be parallel to the mat.

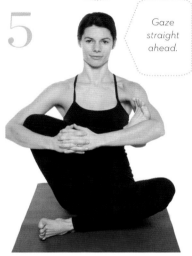

5

Interlace your fingers in front of your leg.

release

To release this pose, simply let go of your leg and find Easy Seat once again.

Peaceful Warrior

Peaceful Warrior is sometimes also called "Reverse Warrior" because it takes the basic shape of our warrior poses and tips the upper body backward in space. Peaceful Warrior strengthens the legs and ankles and allows for a large side stretch from hip to fingertips. Here we practice having open hearts while maintaining stability, feeling like true warriors of peace.

SKILL LEVEL
●●●●○

You can also try lining up your front heel with the back foot's inside arch. See what feels best, then maintain your foundation.

Be sure not to extend your knee over your ankle. Your knee should be placed directly over your ankle.

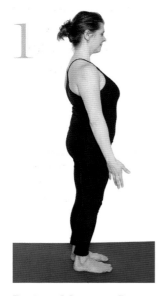 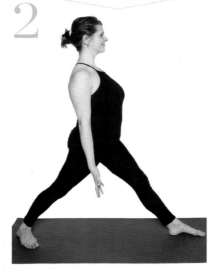 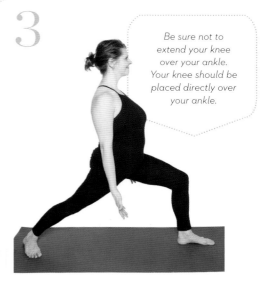

Begin in Mountain Pose, hands out at your sides, feet shoulder-width apart. Feel yourself both rooted into the mat and growing tall in the upper body.

Step your right foot back to a 45 degree angle, so that your front heel lines up with your back heel.

Bend your front leg to a 90 degree angle.

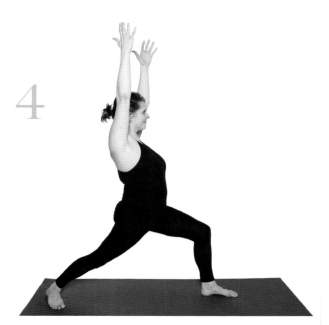

4 Raise your arms overhead keeping them shoulder-width apart.

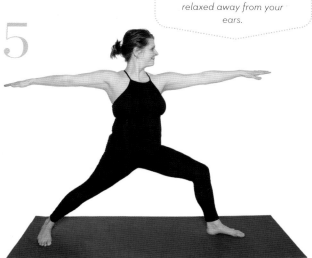

Keep your shoulders relaxed away from your ears.

5 Bring your arms down to shoulder level and extend through your fingers. Open your torso out so your hip bones are now pointing toward the side of the mat.

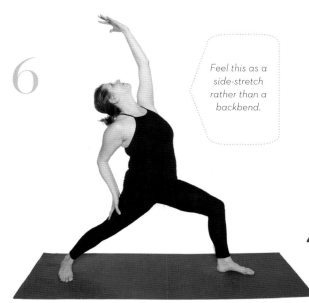

6

Feel this as a side-stretch rather than a backbend.

Take a big breath in, then exhale, reaching the front arm up and slightly back. Allow your back hand to rest lightly on your thigh.

variation

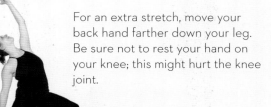

For an extra stretch, move your back hand farther down your leg. Be sure not to rest your hand on your knee; this might hurt the knee joint.

release

To release, move your arms back to straight out and parallel with the floor, bringing the torso upright. From there, bring your arms forward and square your hips to the front of the mat. Then step your feet together into Mountain Pose. Breathe here.

Extended Side Angle

Extended Side Angle Pose (*Utthita Parsvakonasana*) stretches and strengthens the legs and ankles, and stretches the spine, waist, and chest. You'll find extra space in the lungs for deep breaths; this pose often relieves lower back pain as well.

1

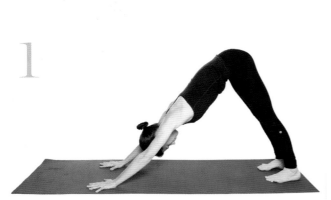

Begin in Downward Facing Dog, hips high and heels reaching toward or pressing into the mat.

2

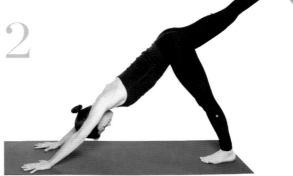

Inhale, then exhale, extending your right leg back and up. Keep your hips square. (If you are a beginner, you can skip this step.)

3

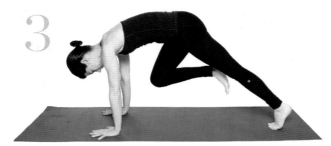

Using your core muscles, step your right foot in between your hands. See if you can step the foot forward lightly. You want to feel your leg is extending from your core, not simply flung into place.

4

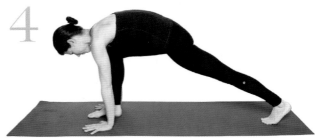

Place your foot so the toes line up with your fingers.

If you feel your back is slouched, bring your right arm up and rest your forearm on your thigh. You can also place a block under the hand that is reaching for the floor. Don't compromise a feeling of lift just for the sake of reaching the ground!

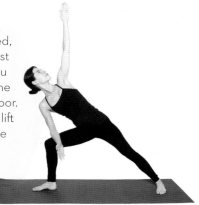

If you're flexible enough, press your palm into the mat.

Strive to spiral the heart and chest upward.

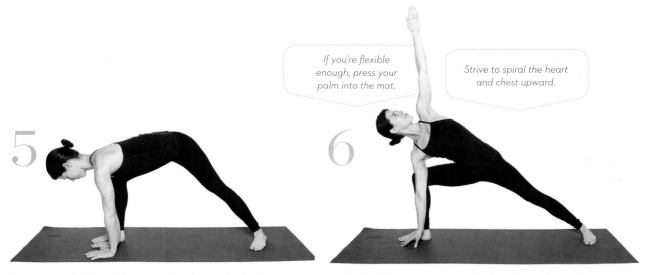

5

Bring your left heel down to the mat with the foot at a 45 degree angle. Lift through your chest, straightening out your back.

6

With the fingers of your right hand touching the earth, bring your left arm up to the sky. Allow the palm of the lifted arm to shine outward. Look up at your fingertips.

release   To release, simply rewind the steps, coming back into Downward Facing Dog. From there you can release into Child's Pose to relax before moving onto the other side.

Pigeon

Pigeon Pose (*Eka Pada Rajakapotasana*) stretches the largest joint in our bodies, the hip joint. This pose also opens the shoulders. You may find emotions arise in this pose, as it's said the hips hold memories and stored emotions. Breathe through any emotions, knowing it's healthy and cleansing to feel and release what was stored inside you! Avoid this pose, or try the variation, if you have any knee pain or a knee or ankle injury.

SKILL LEVEL
● ● ● ● ○

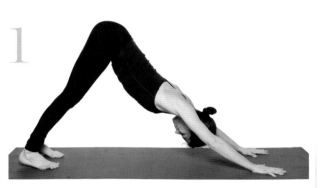

1

Begin in Downward Facing Dog, hips high and heels reaching toward or pressing into the mat.

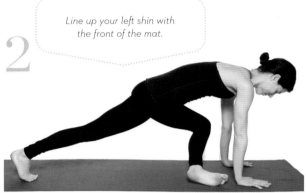

2

Line up your left shin with the front of the mat.

Step your left leg forward, moving your knee to the outside of your left wrist. Flex through your left foot.

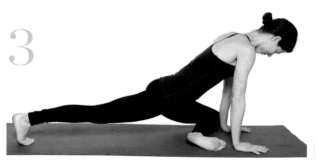

3

To the best of your ability, square your hips toward the mat. Try to move your shin as close to parallel to the front of the mat as possible.

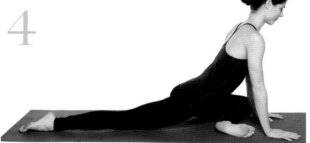

4

Lower your right leg down to the mat to rest, untucking your toes. Square your hips, so the top of your right foot rests on the mat.

Use your breath to help release the hip joint. On each inhale feel space in the heart. On each exhale, sink deeper toward the mat. This pose is largely about letting go, even if things are a little uncomfortable.

keep it easy

If your hip is far from the floor in this posture, try placing a blanket under it.

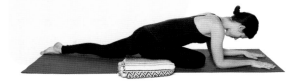

Keep your gaze forward when in this version of Pigeon, with the heart lifted.

5

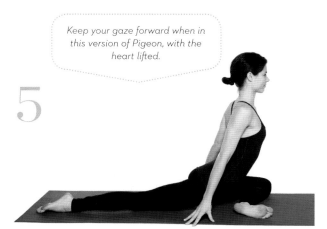

Walk your fingers back toward your hips, stretching and opening up your chest. Feel lift in the heart.

release

To release, press into your hands and transition back into Downward Facing Dog.

flexibility   77

Fish

Fish Pose (*Maysyasana*) stretches the throat, belly, the hip flexors, and even the muscles between the ribs. As the front of the body is stretched, the muscles on the back of the body, specifically the back of the upper back and neck, are strengthened. Even just a few minutes in Fish Pose can leave you feeling energized. It can also be a nice, final heart opener to explore right before resting in Corpse Pose (*Savasana*). Avoid if you have a neck injury.

SKILL LEVEL

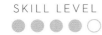

1

Imagine your two legs are fused into a long fish tail.

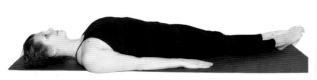

Begin by lying flat on your back with your legs together.

2

Gaze toward your toes.

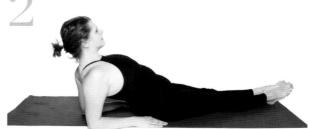

Come up onto your elbows and prop your forearms on the ground. Rest your palms flat with your fingers pointing toward your toes.

You should feel a stretch, but never discomfort or pain in your neck. If you do feel discomfort, move back into step 3 or shift your position so there's less weight on your head and more stretch through the front of your body.

Keep your eyes open and gaze straight ahead.

3

With each inhale, feel the increased expansion in the lungs.

4

For neck safety, it's important not to move your head from side to side. Instead, maintain the connection between the crown of your head and the earth.

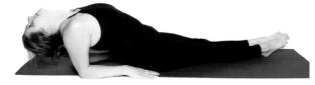

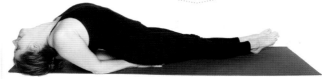

Begin to let your head fall back, opening your heart and throat. This is a wonderful place to stop at first, to feel the stretch in the front of the body.

Move your hands underneath your hips, puffing your chest up further. Allow the crown of your head to rest on the mat.

release   On the exhale, aim to raise your head upright. From there, remove your hands from under your hips. Lie flat on your back.

You must understand the whole of life, not just one little part of it. That is why you must read, that is why you must look at the skies, that is why you must sing, and dance, and write poems, and suffer, and under-stand, for all that is life.

– Jiddu Krishnamurti

BALANCE

The poses in this section will provide opportunities to balance—sometimes on one leg, other times on your toes, or even a knee and a hand! Balancing work in the body does wonders for the mind. It helps us to balance mentally, creating calm concentration.

It's important to approach the challenge of balance with a playful spirit. While the practice of yoga is profound and can create amazing changes in your body, mind, and life, it is also fun and joyful! Keep this in mind especially if you fall out of a balancing shape. Yoga is a practice, not a perfect, and falling out of any pose gives us the opportunity to try, try again. The more we can practice this on the yoga mat the more this spirit of trying again, with a positive approach, will be with us in life, off the mat.

I like to remember the Yoga Sutra, *"Stirum Sukham Asanam,"* which roughly translates to finding a balance of steadiness and ease in poses (and in life!) especially when practicing balancing shapes. A balance of good effort and relaxation exist in all asanas, or poses. In the shapes in this section, see if you can notice where in the body (and mind!) you feel the effort and where you feel the ease. See if you can maintain an equal balance of both qualities.

Another aspect to keep in mind when balancing is where you are looking—in other words, your Gaze, or Drishti. Use your gaze as an anchor when balancing. Keeping a gaze that's both steady and soft can direct focus, translating to a body that's also steady and at ease in the shape.

Above all, enjoy and get curious about how you deal with the challenge of balance. This may give you clues as to how you deal with other challenges in your life off the mat.

Mountain

Mountain Pose (*Tadasana*) firms the legs, ankles, and abdomen while strengthening our connection to the earth. Most of us stand up straight every day, but by fusing this shape with intention and breath we are reminded of the gentle power of a mountain and feel that presence in our own bodies. Practicing Mountain Pose regularly can improve posture and even self-esteem.

SKILL LEVEL
● ○ ○ ○ ○

1

Gaze forward, chin parallel to the mat.

Keep your heart open and your shoulder blades moving back and down. Shoulders melt away from the ears.

2

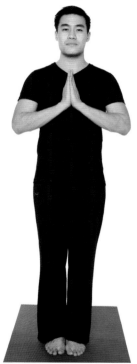

See if you can feel your heart beat against your thumbs.

Stand with your feet together and hands at your side. Try rotating your palms to face forward. Let your fingers gently spread wide with no tension in your hands.

Bring your hands together in front of your heart. Stand quietly. Exhale.

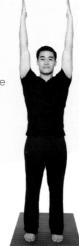

You may prefer to practice Mountain Pose with your feet hip-width apart for a more solid and stable base.

> With each inhale, feel the increased expansion in the lungs.

3

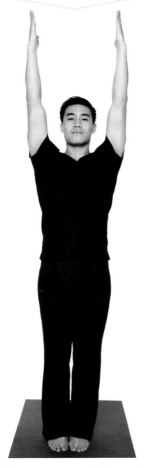

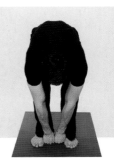

To measure the correct distance of your feet for this variation, bring your hands into fists and place them side by side between your feet.

Take 3 to 5 breaths in this shape, feeling your feet rooting into the earth, your upper body reaching toward the sky. Feel your own shape, both strong and receptive, at ease.

Inhale and bring your arms high overhead. Allow the palms to face each other.

Balancing Tabletop

Balancing Tabletop is sometimes also called Opposite Arm-Leg Extension. This pose strengthens the back muscles and spine and provides a safe way to play with balance. To avoid neck strain, avoid looking upward. Bonus: engaging opposite sides of the body keeps the mind sharp by using both sides of the brain!

SKILL LEVEL
●●○○○

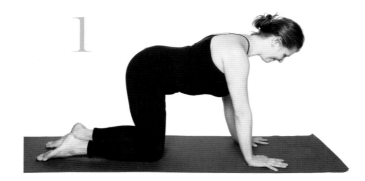

Begin on all fours, making sure your wrists are under your shoulders and your knees under your hips. Gaze straight down with your fingers spread wide.

Think of really engaging your core, pulling the navel toward the spine. It takes belly strength to extend outward.

Try to keep your arm at shoulder height.

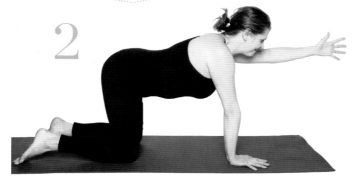

Exhale, then inhale, bringing your left arm straight out in front of you, fingers spread.

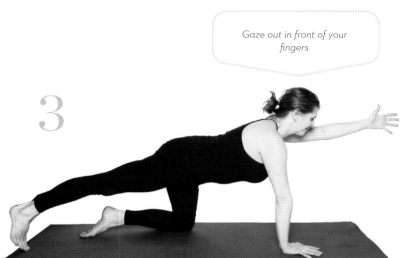

Gaze out in front of your fingers

3

Exhale, then inhale, extending your right leg, keeping your toes pointing downward.

release

To release, exhale both your hand and your knee back down to the mat. It's often nice to practice a few rounds of Cat Pose and Cow Pose following this shape.

Tiptoe Squat

Tiptoe Squat provides a wonderful opportunity to stretch the feet. This can be a particularly potent stretch if you wear heels or walk a lot. This pose also lets us explore balance and mental focus.

SKILL LEVEL
●●●○○

1
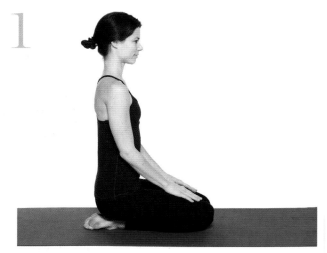
Begin in Hero's Pose, feet tucked under, hands on thighs.

2
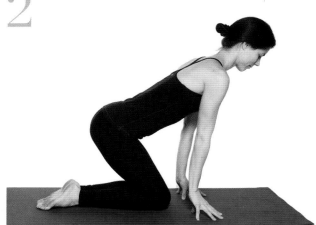
Rock forward, putting your hands on the mat. Tent your fingers and transfer your weight slightly forward.

Use two blocks
under your hands
for balance.

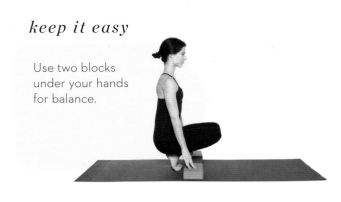

*Think of forming a straight
line, crown of head through
spine to heels.*

3

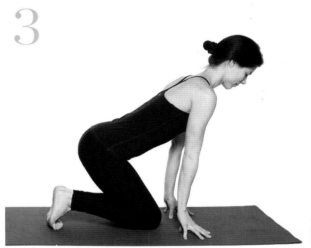

Curl your toes under, keeping weight in your hands.
If you are a beginner, you can stop here. This is
already a strong foot stretch.

4

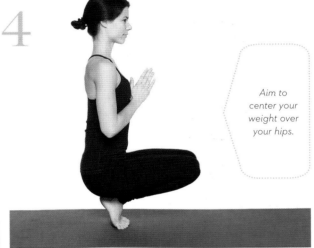

*Aim to
center your
weight over
your hips.*

Shift your weight back and come to balance on your
toes. Bring your hands to heart center in a prayer
position.

release   To release, simply rock your weight forward and come back into Hero's Pose.

Tree

Tree Pose (*Vrksasana*) is a wonderful balancing posture. In this shape we are encouraged to find both steadiness and pliability, just as trees themselves. Tree Pose strengthens the legs and stretches the inner thighs, chest, and shoulders. If you have high blood pressure, avoid raising your arms overhead.

SKILL LEVEL
●●●○○

1
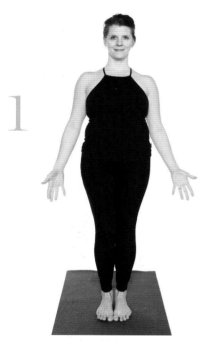

Begin in Mountain Pose with your hands out at your sides.

2
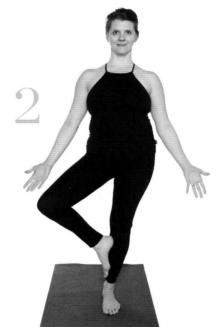

Shift your weight onto your left foot. Move your right foot to your shin and plant the sole of the foot on your calf, with your right knee facing out to the side.

3
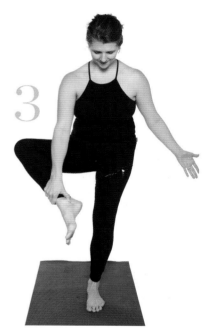

Reach down and grab your right leg at the ankle.

For an additional balance challenge, try closing your eyes. Notice the difference in sensation when sight is out of the picture. Feel how you can keep your balance even with a gentle sway, just as trees do.

keep it easy

For help with balance, keep a chair nearby. Rest one hand lightly on the back of the chair. Try not to lean into the chair, but rather have it there for a little support, keeping your weight in the standing leg. Bring your elevated foot to the calf.

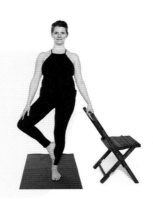

As you practice you'll be able to shift your foot up to the thigh without the help of your hands.

On each inhale feel your heart rising to meet your prayer hands.

Keep your gaze straight ahead.

variation

For an additional balance challenge, straighten out your arms and bring them overhead in a V shape. Palms can face each other or front.

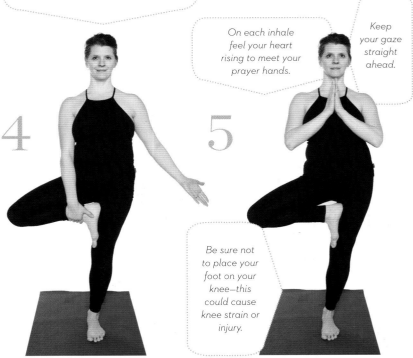

Be sure not to place your foot on your knee—this could cause knee strain or injury.

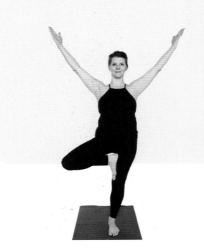

4 Bring the sole of the right foot up to your inner left thigh.

5 Bring your hands together, in front of your heart. Roll your shoulders away from your ears.

release   To release, first allow your arms to drop by your sides. Then mindfully lower the elevated leg. See if you can move out of the shape of tree with grace and balance, too!

Half Moon

Half Moon Pose (*Ardha Chandrasana*) is a wonderful balancing posture that strengthens the legs and opens the heart. This pose can aid digestion and coordination and stretches through the abdomen, legs, chest, and spine. Avoid if you are suffering from a migraine.

SKILL LEVEL
● ● ● ○ ○

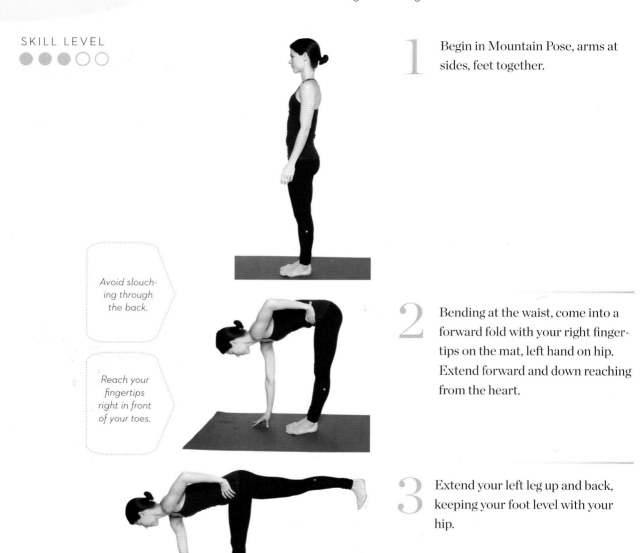

1 Begin in Mountain Pose, arms at sides, feet together.

Avoid slouching through the back.

Reach your fingertips right in front of your toes.

2 Bending at the waist, come into a forward fold with your right fingertips on the mat, left hand on hip. Extend forward and down reaching from the heart.

3 Extend your left leg up and back, keeping your foot level with your hip.

It's more important to feel lift in the heart and extension through both sides of the body than to reach the floor. If you find yourself slumping, use a block under your right hand to raise the floor up to you.

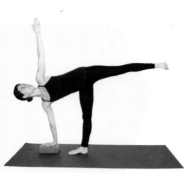

Use your left hand on your hip to "steer" the hip open.

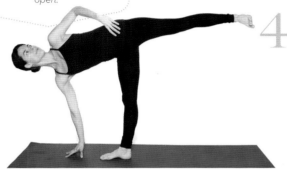

4 Open your hip and torso to the left and look up to the sky.

By keeping your gaze upward you're more likely to keep lift in the shape, an extension upward.

If you have any neck pain or injury, gaze ahead instead of up.

5 Raise your left arm to the sky. Gaze up toward your fingertips.

release

To release, walk through the steps backward. Bring your extended hand back to the mat mindfully, then lower the elevated leg. From here, find a Standing Forward Fold or roll up to stand in Mountain Pose. Feel the effects of Half Moon Pose, then try the other side!

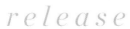

Triangle

Triangle Pose (*Utthita Trikonasana*) works a lot of things at once. In Triangle, you practice balance, strengthen and stretch the legs, and give yourself a large side-stretch from hip to fingertips. Triangle relieves backache, and is an especially great stretch for pregnant yogis.

SKILL LEVEL

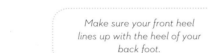

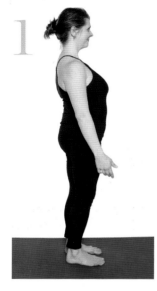

Make sure your front heel lines up with the heel of your back foot.

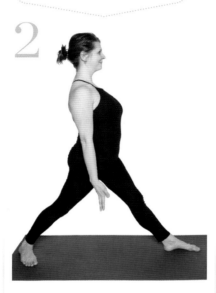

Be sure not to extend your knee over your ankle. Your knee should be placed directly over your ankle.

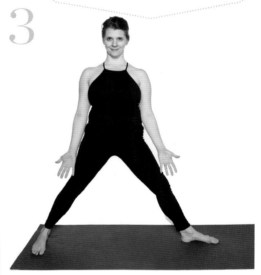

1

Begin in Mountain Pose with your hands by your sides, feet shoulder-width apart.

2

Step back with your right foot and position it at a 45 degree angle, toes pointing to the front corner of the mat.

3

Open your hips to the side, keeping your foot placement.

Think of spiraling the heart open and up toward the sky. The goal is not so much to reach far down on the leg, but to really give yourself a side stretch while rotating your torso upward.

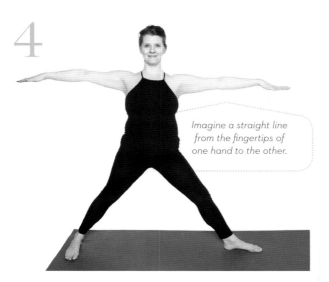

4

Imagine a straight line from the fingertips of one hand to the other.

Bring your arms up to shoulder height, palms facing down.

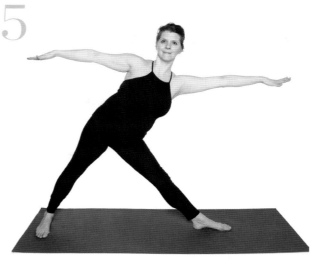

5

Inhale, then exhale and reach out from your hips toward the front of your mat.

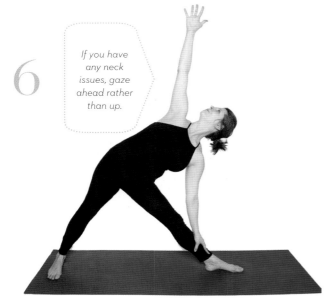

6

If you have any neck issues, gaze ahead rather than up.

Bring your front hand down to rest on your shin. Raise your right hand above your head. Gaze upward.

keep it easy

Use a block for your front hand, or …

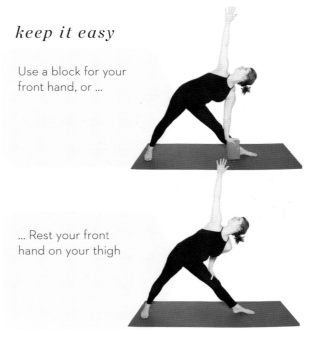

… Rest your front hand on your thigh

release

To release the pose, reverse the steps. Walk your lowered fingertips up your leg and find your wide-legged stance with arms extended. From there, lower your arms and step back up into Mountain Pose. Be sure to do Triangle Pose on both sides!

Dancer's Pose

Dancer's Pose (*Natarajasana*) is a beautiful balancing posture. Here you will strengthen the standing leg while stretching through the thighs, chest, and shoulders. Dancer's Pose also encourages mental focus and grace!

SKILL LEVEL
●●●●○

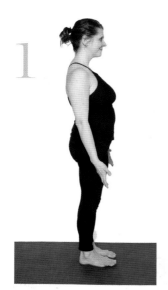
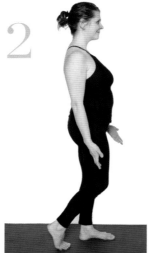
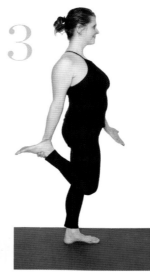
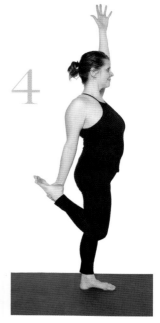

1	2	3	4
Begin in Mountain Pose, hands out at your sides, feet shoulder-width apart.	Shift your weight into your left foot. Bring your right foot back a bit.	Reach down with your right hand and grab your right foot from the inside. Allow the palm of your left hand to face forward or toward the right.	Inhale, then exhale, reaching up to the sky with your left hand. Spread your fingers wide.

Use a chair for balance. Gaze ahead. Feel the press of your foot into your hand moving you forward in space with the chair there to support you.

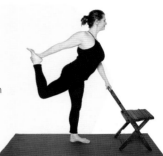

With each inhale think of growing longer. With each exhale, tip a little further forward.

Try a mudra with your left hand.

5

Gaze ahead. If you look down, you may tip down!

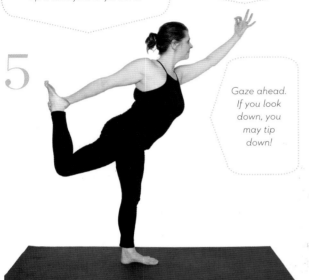

6

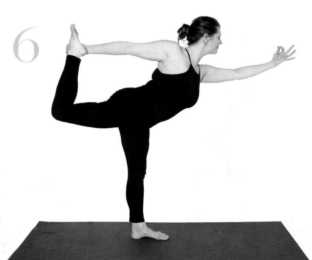

Begin to extend with your right leg, pressing into your right hand with your right foot. Bend forward, reaching outward.

Lean forward more. Think of squaring your hips toward the floor. Imagine there's a straight line from your front fingers to your back foot.

release

To release, take a big breath in, then exhale and, keeping the hold on your foot, come back to standing upright. Inhale, then exhale, releasing your foot. Stand in Mountain Pose.

Eagle

Eagle Pose (*Garudasana*), is actually named after the Garuda, a mythic "king of the birds." This posture improves our balance and concentration; strengthens the legs; and stretches the hips, shoulders, and upper back. Yogis with knee injuries should practice this pose with only the upper body, or in single leg wrap as described in Step 3.

SKILL LEVEL
●●●●○

> Make sure your knees are over your ankles. Don't let them go out in front of your toes.

> Your gaze can be a helpful tool here. By gazing at one point you improve your focus and aid balance.

1

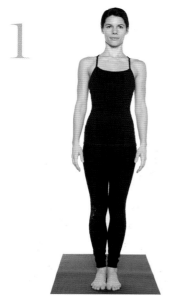

Begin in Mountain Pose, feet together.

2

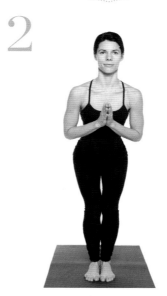

Bring your hands to your heart, and sit down and back as if in a little chair.

3

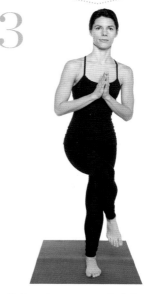

Balancing on your left foot, bring your right leg up and wrap it around your left. Try to bring the right leg as high up as possible on the left leg so you have more room to wrap.

If you have tight shoulders and find the arm wrap very challenging, just hug each shoulder with the opposite hand. This has the same effect, stretching the upper back and shoulders.

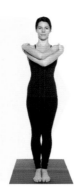

4

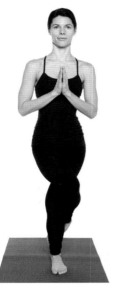

Wrap your foot behind your leg (Beginners can leave this step out, and just wrap the leg, not the foot.)

5

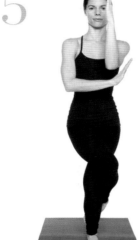

Try to elevate your elbows so your hands are at eye level.

Bring your left arm up, and move your right arm under your left.

6

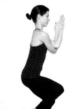

Close-up of the hand position.

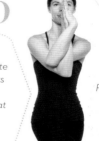

Final pose from the side.

Line up your elbows, and press your palms together.

release   To release, slowly unwind your legs and come to stand. Then, unwind your arms, finding Mountain Pose.

Warrior 3

Warrior 3 (*Virabhadrasana III*) is indeed a fierce warrior pose, cultivating strength, balance, and bravery. Here we strengthen the legs and ankles along with the muscles of the back. We also improve balance. Move carefully or avoid if you have high blood pressure.

SKILL LEVEL

●●●●○

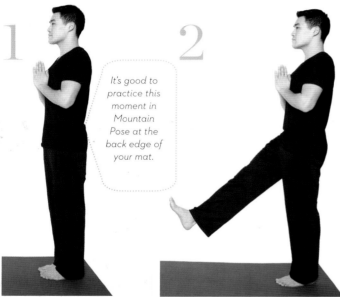

It's good to practice this moment in Mountain Pose at the back edge of your mat.

1 Begin in Mountain Pose, hands pressed together in front of your heart. Inhale.

2 Exhale, and extend your right leg forward as if taking a big step.

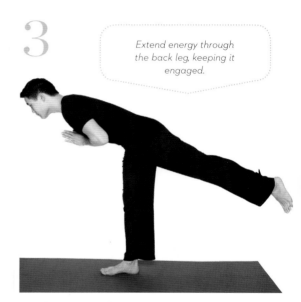

Extend energy through the back leg, keeping it engaged.

3 Rock your weight forward, transferring your weight to your right foot. Extend your left leg back.

variation

For another variation, extend your arms back, palms down. This is often called Airplane Variation.

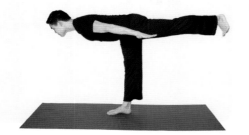

keep it easy

Use a chair to help with your balance. Place the chair far enough in front of you so your arms and back leg can extend, finding the letter T shape in your body.

4

Imagine a straight line of energy running from the top of your head through your back foot.

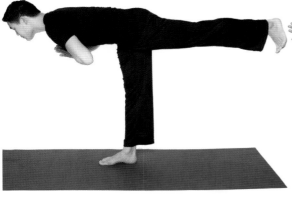

Begin to shift your weight forward so your left leg is as close to parallel with the mat as possible. (This is a fine place to stop for beginners.)

5

Imagine you are a capital letter T.

Gaze slightly forward and down. Try not to let your neck get strained up or down.

For added challenge, extend your arms out in front, palms facing one another, fingers spread.

release Simply rock your weight backward, bringing the extended leg to the mat. Step on this foot and bring both feet together. Rest in Mountain Pose before trying the other side.

Standing Split

Standing Split (*Urdhva Prasarita Eka Padasana*) is a fun inversion and balancing posture. It's known to calm the mind; stretch the back of the leg, front of the thigh, and groin; and strengthen the standing leg all at once. Avoid if you have a knee or lower back injury.

As with many yoga poses, there is no set goal or "place to be." It's wonderful to stop at any of these steps. Step 3, with hands on the floor, may be your Standing Split today. With time, or on a different day, you may enjoy step 7, the "no hands" version.

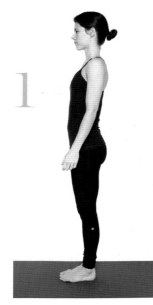

1

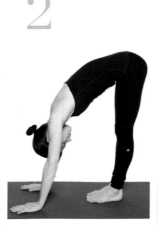

2

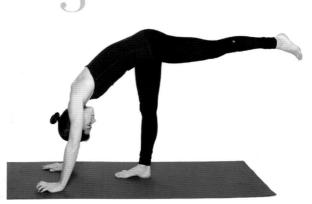

3

Begin in Mountain Pose, feet together.

Fold forward at the waist, bringing your hands to the mat. Drop your head.

Put your weight in your right foot, and begin to slowly bring up the left. Keep your left leg parallel to the mat at first, hips square. Allow your head to drop and your back to be as relaxed as possible.

4

Walk your right hand back so it lines up with your heel.

keep it easy

Try using two blocks under your hands for balance and to bring the floor up to you. From here, you can drop your upper body, shifting the blocks back in space with you, and coming further into your Standing Split with the blocks.

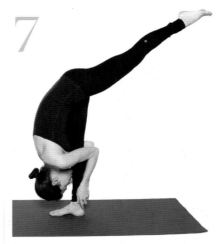

5

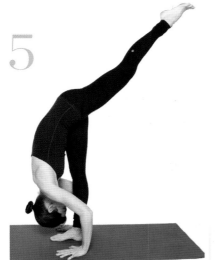

Bring your left hand back to align with your right. Allow your upper body to tip further forward. (If you're a beginner, you can stop here.)

6

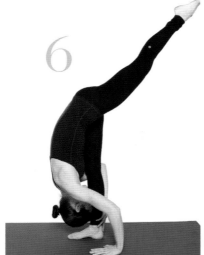

Extend your left leg higher, if you can. Bring your right forearm behind your right calf.

7

Bring both hands to the standing leg's calf or ankle.

release   To release, simply walk backward through the steps, coming into a forward fold, then rolling up to stand.

To be nobody but yourself in a world which is doing its best, night and day, to make you everybody else means to fight the hardest battle which any human being can fight; and never stop fighting.

-e. e. cummings

STRENGTH

One of the gifts of yoga is increased strength. The poses in this section build strength in different parts of the body such as the core, the legs, and the arms. Through yoga practice you'll develop a well-balanced strength throughout the entire body. There is no need to feel strong from the get-go when you try these postures. The poses will work with your body and will meet you where you are now. From this honest starting point, anyone can build strength.

In working on these strengthening poses, see if you can practice "finding your edge." Challenge yourself and don't be afraid of the feeling of new muscles growing, and the effort that comes with it. But never work into pain! You do want to feel challenged, but if you ever start to feel pain in a pose, back out and rest.

One of the wonderful things about building strength through yoga is that you don't need any weights, machines, or contraptions. You only need your body, breath, intention, and willing spirit. See if you can keep your inhales and exhales even throughout unless otherwise noted. If your breath ever begins to grow labored or short, that may be the body's way of telling you it's time to rest.

Strength built through yoga will lead to a lean, capable body; increased confidence; and sense of self. Yoga strength is paired with flexibility: usually when you are strengthening one thing in a pose you are actually stretching another! (Poses are brilliant that way.) Strength built through yoga will not make you bulky. If anything, you are fine-tuning the instrument of your body and growing strong and capable in mind and spirit. You will grow capable in moving assuredly through space.

Superhero

Superhero (*Salabhasana*) is a variation of Locust Pose, as the Sanskit translates to. This pose is a wonderful and safe back strengthener. It will improve your posture, ease and prevent lower back pain, stimulate digestion, and help remove stress. Plus, you're taking on the shape of a superhero flying over cities with a cape! Feel your own super powers.

SKILL LEVEL

●●○○○

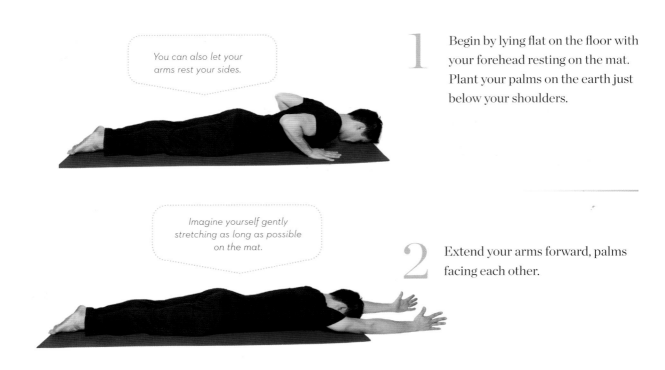

You can also let your arms rest your sides.

1 Begin by lying flat on the floor with your forehead resting on the mat. Plant your palms on the earth just below your shoulders.

Imagine yourself gently stretching as long as possible on the mat.

2 Extend your arms forward, palms facing each other.

This is a full *pranam,* or prostration. It can be felt as a gesture of surrender. Let yourself be held by the earth.

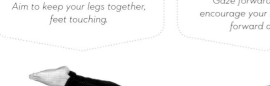

Aim to keep your legs together, feet touching.

Gaze forward and up to encourage your body to move forward and up.

3 Inhale then exhale, raising your arms, chest, and legs off the mat.

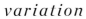

variation

Move your arms back, palms facing the mat. Keep your arms by your sides. With each inhale, imagine your feet and upper body elevating further. With each exhale, think of lengthening head to toe.

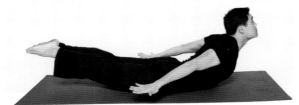

release

Release on an exhale, slowly lowering your body to the mat.

strength   105

Boat

Boat Pose (*Navasana*) is a wonderful core strengthener, touching upon the abdomen, hip flexors, and spine. And, as we know, a strong core is the key to a strong back! Boat Pose also encourages balance and mental focus.

SKILL LEVEL
● ● ● ○ ○

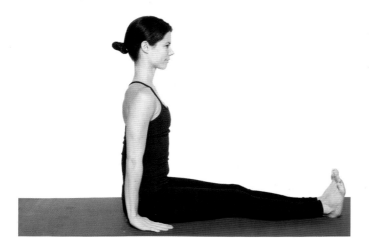

1 Begin in Staff Pose, legs straight on the floor and glued together as if you have one long leg. Flex your feet so toes point up and back.

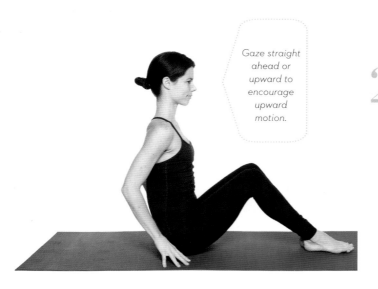

Gaze straight ahead or upward to encourage upward motion.

2 Walk your toes back to bring your knees up. Place your feet flat on the floor, fingers tented beside your hips.

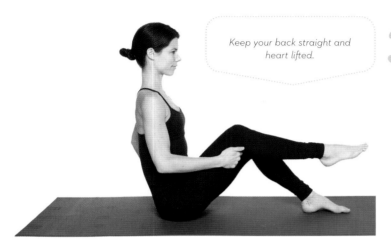

Keep your back straight and heart lifted.

3 Using a hand under your thigh, bring your right leg up.

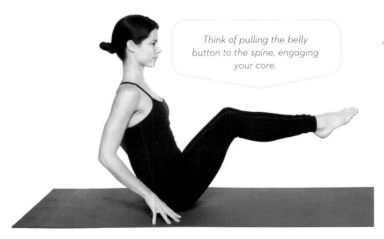

Think of pulling the belly button to the spine, engaging your core.

4 Bring your left leg up to meet your right. Place your tented fingers next to your hips.

release   To release, simply walk backward through these steps, coming into Staff Pose.

Plank

Plank Pose strengthens the arms, legs, wrists, and core. Your entire body will be engaged with firm energy.

SKILL LEVEL

Make sure your hands are directly under your shoulders, fingers spread wide.

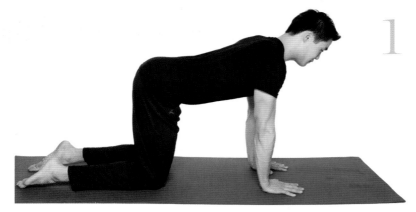

1   Begin on all fours. Gaze down.

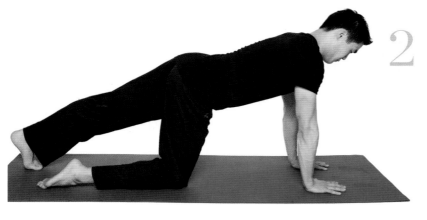

2   Step back with your left leg, toes tucked under.

If you have carpal tunnel syndrome or any wrist pain, consider practicing on your forearms, in a Forearm Plank.

Come down onto your knees, with your legs bent. Allow your knees on the mat to provide extra support. Still think of keeping your tailbone tucked, core engaged.

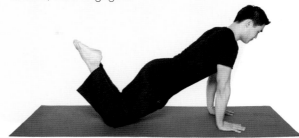

It is common for your hips to rise here. Be sure to tuck your tailbone and think of pulling your belly button toward your spine to keep your body in a straight line.

3   Step back with your right leg, toes tucked under.

Gaze downward and a little in front of your fingers to keep your neck neutral.

Think of pushing energy out your heels, engaging the body from the top of the head through the feet.

release   To release, slowly lower your body down to the mat. You can also lower your knees first, then push back to a Child's Pose.

strength   109

Chaturanga

Chaturanga (*Chaturanga Dandasana*) is a very strengthening posture for the arms, wrists, and core of the body. It is usually a transitional posture between Plank Pose and Upward Facing Dog. Proceed carefully if you have carpal tunnel syndrome or other wrist pain.

SKILL LEVEL
●●●○○

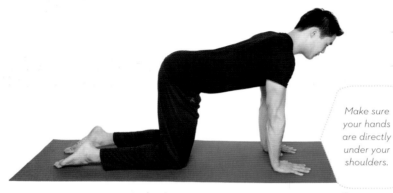

1 Begin on all fours, fingers spread wide. Gaze downward.

Make sure your hands are directly under your shoulders.

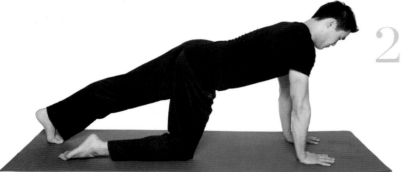

2 Step back with your left leg, toes tucked under.

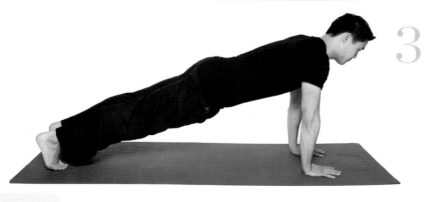

3 Step back with your right leg, toes tucked under. Here you are in Plank Pose.

keep it easy

Come down onto your knees, with your legs bent. Allow your knees on the mat to provide extra support.

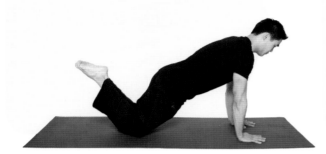

Still think of keeping your tailbone tucked, core engaged.

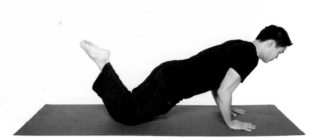

Really think of using your core muscles, tucking your tailbone slightly, to support the shape.

4 Lower yourself down until your elbows are at a 90 degree angle.

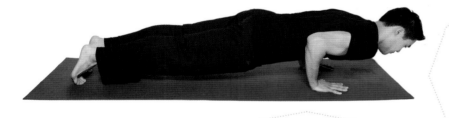

Gaze down to keep your neck in a neutral position.

Make sure your elbows are pointing back toward your feet.

release   To release, either push back up to a Plank Pose or lower slowly onto your belly. Note that Chaturanga often leads into Upward Facing Dog, so that is a good transition to practice as well.

Chair

Chair Pose (*Utkatasana*) is all about strength! In Sanskrit the pose translates to "powerful, fierce" pose. Through Chair Pose you'll build strength in the legs, spine, and core, and will both activate and stretch the arms and shoulders. Get ready to feel powerful!

SKILL LEVEL
●●●○○

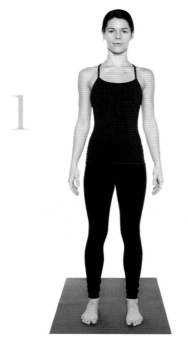

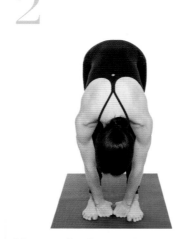

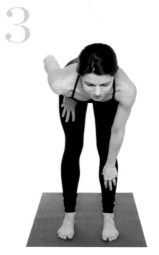

1

Begin in Mountain Pose, arms at your sides, and feet shoulder-width apart.

2

Measure the distance between your legs by placing your fists together between your feet. That's your hip distance.

3

Come up to standing, walking your hands up your legs. Pull your belly button toward your spine and feel your lower belly engaged to protect your back.

The wonderful thing about Chair Pose is you control how far down you sit. To keep things easy, sit down less, keeping a smaller bend in the knees. Over time you'll want to sit down deeper.

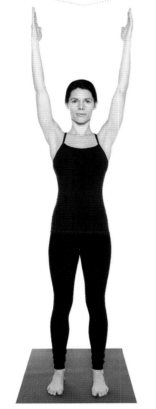

Relax your shoulders away from your ears as much as possible.

4

Raise your arms overhead, palms facing inward.

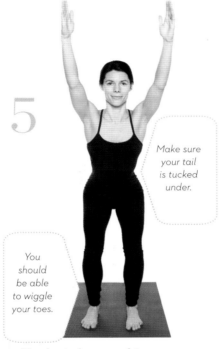

Be sure your knees are over your ankles, to protect the knee joints.

5

Make sure your tail is tucked under.

You should be able to wiggle your toes.

Slowly sit down, making sure your weight is in your heels. Pretend you're sitting in a little child's chair.

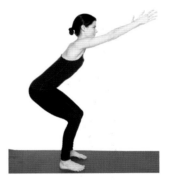

Final pose from the side.

To feel the effects of Chair Pose, stay for around 5 breaths. With each inhale reach further up with your arms and feel lift in the chest. With each exhale, sit further back and down, being sure your knees aren't poking forward over your ankles.

release   On an exhale, push up to stand, finding your Mountain Pose. Allow your arms to rest by your sides, feeling the effects of the pose.

High Lunge

High Lunge is sometimes also referred to as Crescent Lunge. In this pose we cultivate mental and physical focus and balance. This posture strengthens the legs and core, stretches the upper back and chest, and improves posture.

SKILL LEVEL
●●●○○

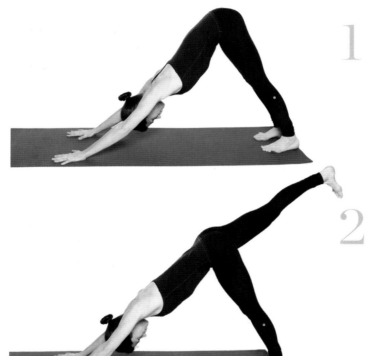

1   Begin in Downward Facing Dog.

2   Inhale, bringing your right leg back and up. (You can skip this step if you are a beginner.)

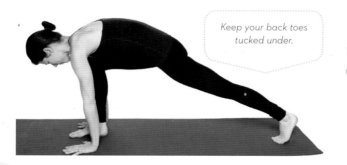

Keep your back toes tucked under.

3   Exhale, stepping your right foot in between your hands. See if you can line up fingertips and toes.

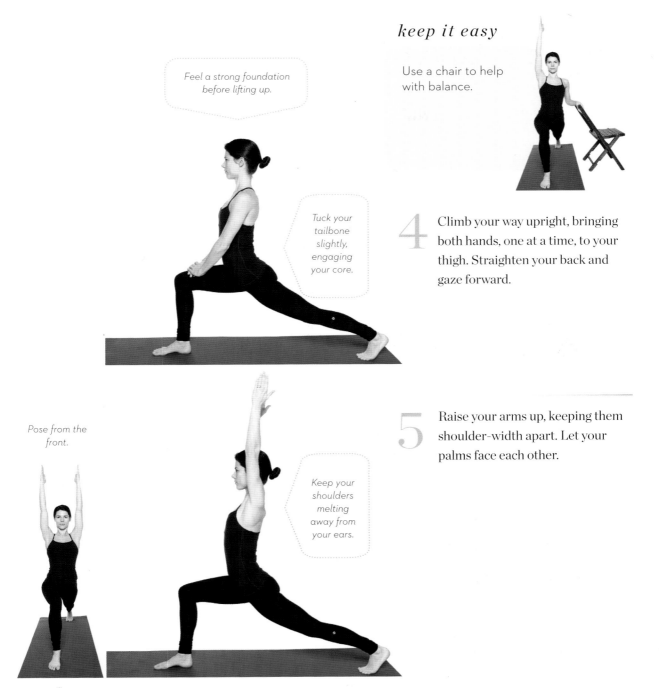

Feel a strong foundation before lifting up.

Use a chair to help with balance.

Tuck your tailbone slightly, engaging your core.

4 Climb your way upright, bringing both hands, one at a time, to your thigh. Straighten your back and gaze forward.

5 Raise your arms up, keeping them shoulder-width apart. Let your palms face each other.

Pose from the front.

Keep your shoulders melting away from your ears.

release

On an exhale, bring your hands down to the mat on either side of your front foot. Take a big breath in, then step back to Downward Facing Dog. From here, you can rest in Child's Pose before trying the other foot.

Warrior 1

Warrior 1 (*Virabhadrasana I*) is a strong posture that cultivates the feeling of a peaceful warrior from the inside out. This pose strengthens and stretches the legs, feet, and ankles, as well as the shoulders, arms, and back. You will feel expansion in the lungs and chest and heat in the legs as you create strength and space. In this pose we practice embodying a strong stable peace. See if you can feel that quality even in your gaze.

SKILL LEVEL
● ● ● ○ ○

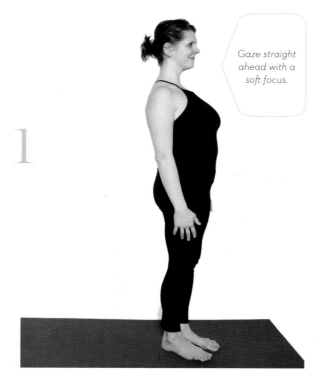

Gaze straight ahead with a soft focus.

1

Begin in Mountain Pose, hands out at your sides, feet shoulder-width apart.

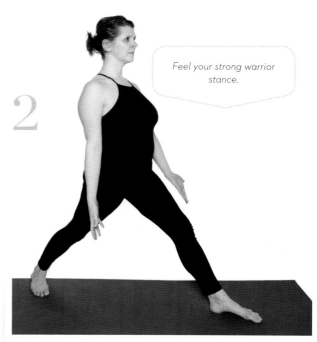

Feel your strong warrior stance.

2

Step your right foot back at 45 degree angle, so your front heel lines up with your back heel.

variation

Press your palms together overhead, continuing to keep your shoulders away from your ears. People with shoulder issues may prefer the arms shoulder-width apart.

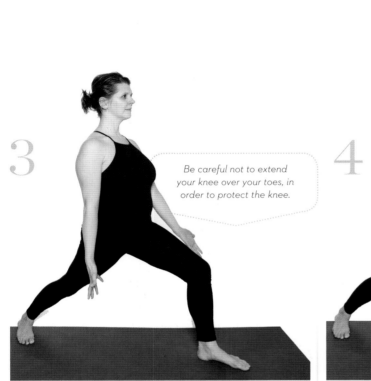

3

Be careful not to extend your knee over your toes, in order to protect the knee.

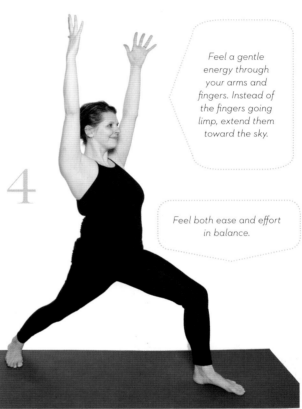

4

Feel a gentle energy through your arms and fingers. Instead of the fingers going limp, extend them toward the sky.

Feel both ease and effort in balance.

Bend your front leg to a 90 degree angle so your thigh is parallel to the earth.

Raise your hands overhead. On each inhale, feel extra space in your lungs and within the shape. On each exhale, sink a little lower, being sure to keep your knee over your ankle. Smile and stay for 3 to 5 breaths.

release   To release the pose, rewind the steps, coming back into Mountain Pose. Be sure to do the other side!

strength   117

Warrior 2

Warrior II (*Virabhadrasana II*) allows us to feel strong, stable, and open-hearted at the same time. This pose gives us permission to take up space. You're encouraged to stretch from fingertip to fingertip, through the hips and legs. This pose stretches and strengthens the legs, ankles, chest, and shoulders, and can relieve backaches. It's also a safe way to stretch and relieve back pain for pregnant yogis.

SKILL LEVEL
● ● ● ○ ○

Be careful not to extend your knee over your toes, in order to protect the knee.

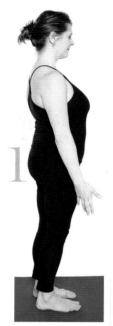

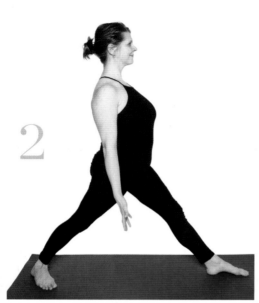

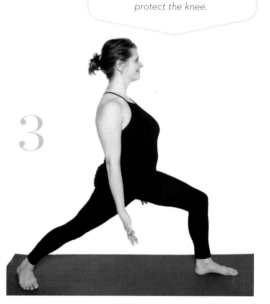

Begin in Mountain Pose, hands out at your sides, feet shoulder-width apart.

Step your right foot back to a 45 degree angle, so your front heel lines up with your back heel.

Bend your front leg to a 90 degree angle.

variation

Lining up heels allows for a wider stance. For a different feeling and more of a balance challenge, try lining up your front heel with the inside arch of your back foot.

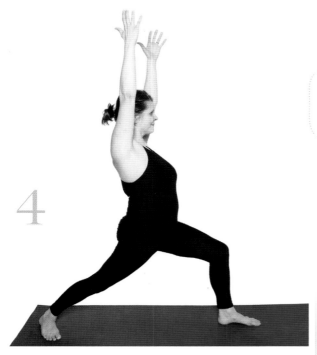

4

Raise your arms overhead on an inhale. (You'll be in Warrior I for a moment.)

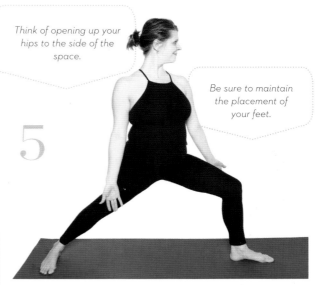

Think of opening up your hips to the side of the space.

Be sure to maintain the placement of your feet.

5

Bring your arms down and turn your torso out.

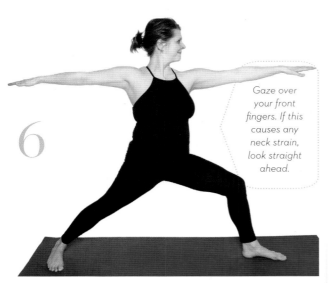

Gaze over your front fingers. If this causes any neck strain, look straight ahead.

6

Extend your arms up to shoulder level. Reach gently through your fingers. Imagine one line of energy running from the fingertips of one hand through to the fingertips of the other hand.

With each inhale, imagine you are growing wider and larger. With each exhale, sink further down in your lunge, being careful not to extend your front knee over your ankle.

release

To release, simply walk yourself through the steps in reverse. It's nice to bring your arms up by your ears and square your hips to the front of the mat, visiting Warrior I for a moment once again. From there, step your back foot in and find Mountain Pose to finish.

Side Plank

Side Plank (*Vasisthasana*) is a balancing pose that strengthens the core of the body, the arms, and the legs. Move into this shape carefully or avoid if you have a shoulder or wrist injury.

SKILL LEVEL

● ● ● ● ○

The hips sometimes have the tendency to dip in this shape. With each exhale, think of raising your hips and side body further toward the ceiling. Feel the energy engaging all parts of your body, fingers to toes!

1

Gaze downward.

Spread your fingers wide.

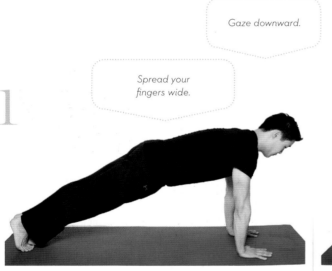

Begin in Plank Pose, shoulders and wrists aligned, your core engaged.

2

Imagine you have one line of energy running from the top of your head through your heels.

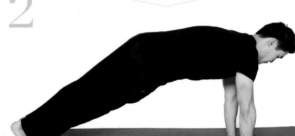

Bring your left hand to the center of the mat, directly under your heart.

keep it easy

If you are finding it hard to maintain balance, bring your left knee to the mat. In this position, line up your bent knee with your toes so you form a triangle shape with both legs.

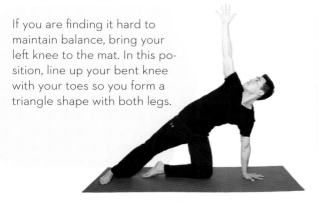

You can also keep your bottom leg straight while crossing your top leg over with knee bent. Plant your right foot on the ground. Keep pushing your hips upward!

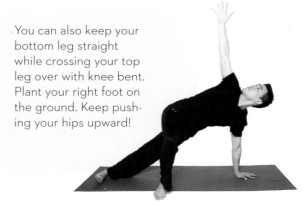

Gaze up toward your fingertips.

3

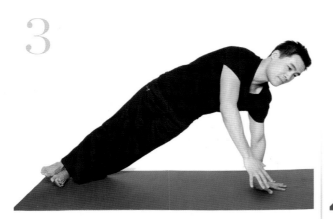

Begin to shift your weight so you stack your feet one on top of the other. Press into the earth with your left hand.

4

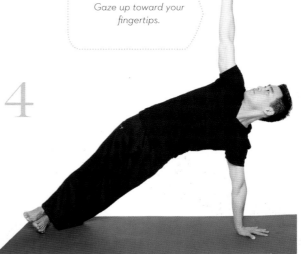

Bring your right arm up to the sky, pushing your hips to the ceiling.

release   To release, simply move back into Plank Pose. From there, move to the other side. To rest, come into Child's Pose or lower onto your belly.

Dolphin

Dolphin Pose is a wonderful shape that strengthens the arms, legs, and shoulders while stretching through the hamstrings and calves. The inversion aspect also calms the mind and lightens mild depression. Dolphin is a great preparatory pose if you plan to try arm balances. Proceed carefully if you have a shoulder injury.

SKILL LEVEL

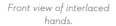

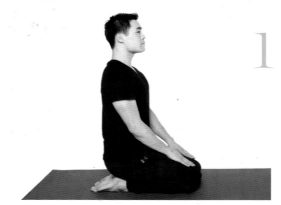

1 Begin in Hero's Pose, palms resting on your thighs.

Front view of interlaced hands.

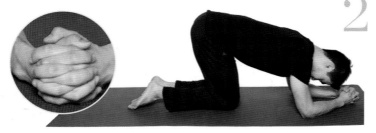

2 Come forward and place your elbows on the mat. Interlace the fingers of your hands creating a tripod shape with your hands, forearms, and elbows.

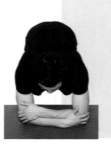

You can measure the shape between your elbows by unlacing your fingers and reaching for your elbows with opposite hands. Your right fingertips should reach the outside of your left elbow. Your left fingertips should reach the outside of your right elbow.

keeping it easy

For more support, extend your forearms parallel on the mat, fingers splayed out wide. This is good if you have a wrist injury.

For an easier way to come up into Downward Facing Dog, just curl your toes under on both feet and lift up from there.

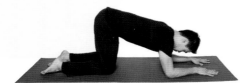

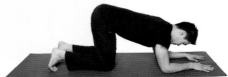

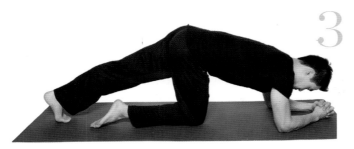

3 Extend your left leg. Bend your toes under on the mat.

Push into the mat with your elbows to make sure you aren't scrunched through the shoulders. You want to feel your shoulders are moving away from your ears.

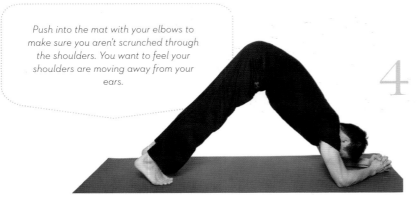

4 Extend your right leg back, toes tucked under. Bring your hips up into Downward Facing Dog. Let your head drop.

release To release, mindfully bend your knees down to the mat. Push back into Child's Pose.

Be really whole,

And all things will come

to you.

-Tao Te Ching

RESTORATIVE

Restorative poses allow the body, mind, and spirit a chance to deeply rest and, indeed, restore. In our fast-paced modern world with our over-active lifestyles, it's important to make the time for rest. For many of us this can be a rather challenging part of yoga practice. If you are used to going full speed, multitasking and emphasizing accomplishment even in exercise, it can be hard to relax, slow down, and just *be*. Know that restoration is actually very productive. Without this part of our yoga practice we would not have time to allow the benefits of the more active yoga poses to sink in. We would not have time to reflect. Restorative poses also allow us opportunities to meditatively watch the mind.

If time allows, stay in these poses for many long deep breaths or minutes. Corpse Pose (*Savasana*) is included in this section and often is the last pose of yoga practices. With this posture you'll want to stay and explore the shape for up to 15 minutes.

Much of our yoga practice falls on the "yang" side of things—yang meaning more active, dynamic. The poses in the restorative section lean more toward the "yin," meaning softer, more receptive, relaxing. This does not mean these poses are passive in any way. In fact, as you settle into the restorative poses in this section, trust that they benefit mind, body, and breath.

In yoga we hope to be fully active when it's active time and fully relaxed when it's time to relax. Part of our practice is honoring both states!

Legs Up the Wall

Legs Up the Wall (*Viparita Karani*) is a very powerful pose that should be practiced often. This pose relieves many things such as anxiety, digestive issues, arthritis, headaches, menstrual cramps, and varicose veins. It is even said to be anti-aging. Be careful or skip if you have serious back issues that could be aggravated by this pose.

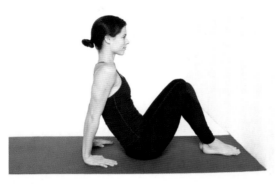

1 Sit on the floor, knees up, hands behind you, toes near the wall.

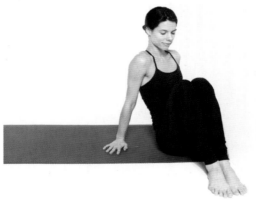

2 Slide closer to the wall, bringing your bottom to touch the wall, both legs to one side.

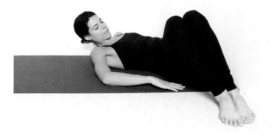

3 Lean back on your elbows and move your bottom close to the wall.

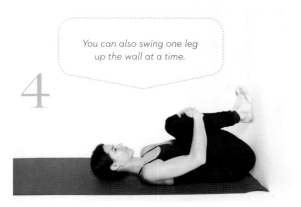

You can also swing one leg up the wall at a time.

4

Lay on your back, bottom against the wall, and place both feet on the wall.

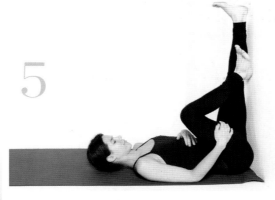

5

Straighten out your left leg.

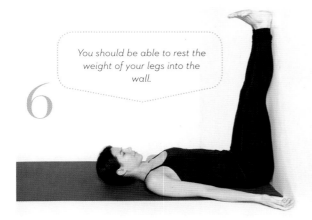

You should be able to rest the weight of your legs into the wall.

6

Straighten out your right leg. Move your bottom as close to the wall as possible, or touching.

keep it easy

If your feet start to feel too tingly, try pressing the soles of your feet together, letting your knees flop open into a butterfly shape. Then, allow your feet to drop down the wall, closer to your bottom.

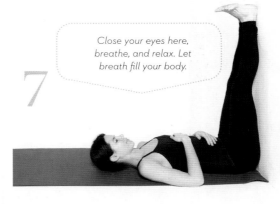

Close your eyes here, breathe, and relax. Let breath fill your body.

7

Place your right hand on your belly, your left hand on your heart; or place your hands by your sides. Stay in this pose for 5 to 15 minutes.

release

To release, bend your knees, placing the soles of your feet on the wall. Then, turn onto your right side, bringing your legs with you. Slowly roll up to a seated posture.

Corpse

Corpse Pose (*Savasana*) is a full-body resting pose that usually happens at the end of yoga practice. Though it may look like simply lying on the floor, with the power of intention and breath this pose can be infused with meaning. Here, our bodies, minds, and spirits have a chance to soak up all the benefits of the postures that came before. Corpse Pose calms the mind and can lower blood pressure.

SKILL LEVEL
● ○ ○ ○ ○

Allow your body to be heavy and your mind to be light. Feel as if you're melting into the floor.

1 Lay down with your arms at your sides. Let your legs fall open. Imagine there's a center line running down your body and your arms and legs are flopping symmetrically open from it. Stay in this pose for 5 to 15 minutes.

For many yogis, it can be more challenging to lie still and relax than to move through poses. Recognize the challenge if this resonates with you.

keep it easy

If you have any discomfort in your lower back, place a rolled-up blanket under your knees for lift and support.

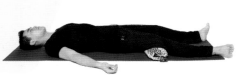

If any thoughts or worries arise in the mind, see if you can notice them but then redirect your attention back to gentle, natural breathing and the intention of letting go. Corpse Pose is where we practice letting go.

release To release, roll slowly onto the right side of your body. Stay there, curled in the fetal position, for several breaths. Then, place your left hand to the earth and gently push up to sit.

Half Happy Baby

Half Happy Baby is just that, half of a Happy Baby Pose. Here we focus on one leg and one hip joint at a time. This pose stretches the groin and large joint of the hip. Stay in the shape for several breaths. With each exhale, think of melting further into the mat.

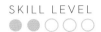

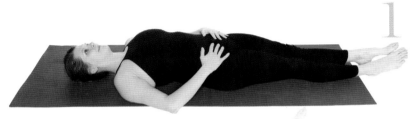

1 Lay flat on the floor allowing your hands to rest on your lower belly or hips. Feel yourself grounded on the earth.

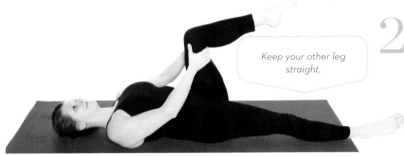

Keep your other leg straight.

2 Reach with both hands for the bottom of your left thigh. Gently bring your knee in toward your chest.

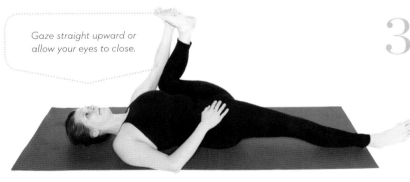

Gaze straight upward or allow your eyes to close.

3 Keep your right hand on your right hip to ground it. With your left hand, grab the outside of your left foot. Draw your left knee into your armpit.

release   Release your lifted foot. Allow your legs to come out straight, resting on the floor.

restorative   129

Happy Baby

Happy Baby (*Ananda Balasana*) got its name from babies, who often fall naturally into this shape. This posture stretches and releases both hips at the same time, plus stretches the groin and the lower back. Happy Baby also calms the mind, relieving stress to help us be happy. Proceed gently if you have any knee or neck injuries; listen to your body.

SKILL LEVEL
●●○○○

Feel the support of the earth under you.

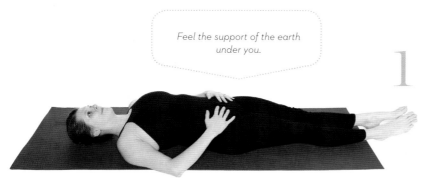

1 Begin by lying flat on the floor, hands on your lower abdomen or hips.

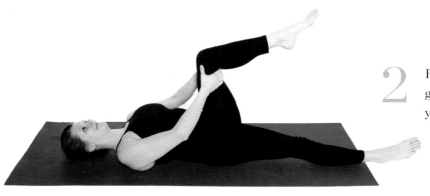

2 Reach down with both hands and gently pull your left knee toward your chest.

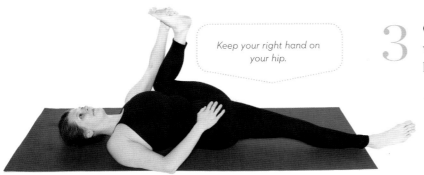

Keep your right hand on your hip.

3 Grab the outside of your left foot with your left hand, drawing your knee into your armpit.

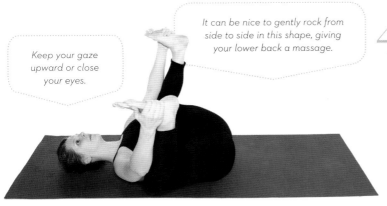

Keep your gaze upward or close your eyes.

It can be nice to gently rock from side to side in this shape, giving your lower back a massage.

4 Draw your right knee into and outside of your chest, toward your armpit. Allow your right hand to hold the outside of your foot.

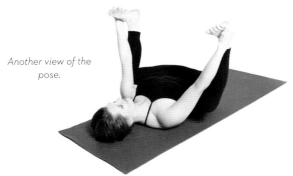

Another view of the pose.

This is a great pose to try Lion's Breath in. Take a big breath in the nose, then exhale out the mouth, sticking out your tongue. It may feel silly, but no one can see, and it's a great way to release stress, leaving you like a happy baby!

release To release, let go of your feet and bring the soles of your feet to the mat. Feel free to windshield-wiper your knees back and forth to release your back.

Standing Forward Fold

Standing Forward Fold (*Uttanasana*) calms the mind, eases mild depression, and improves digestion while stretching the back of the legs and the hips. It is very powerful to drop the head below the heart this way and allow the spine to decompress in a forward fold! If you feel any back discomfort or have a back injury, try with bent knees.

SKILL LEVEL
●●○○○

1
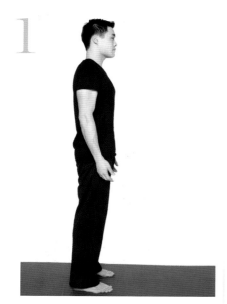

Begin in Mountain Pose, hands at your sides, palms facing forward.

2

Keep your neck soft. Shake your head "yes" and "no" to release any stubborn tension.

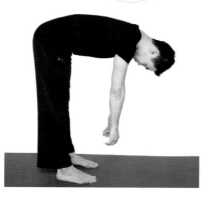

Inhale, then exhale, beginning to bend from the hips, releasing your upper body forward and down. Let your arms hang and your head drop.

3

It doesn't matter if your hands reach the floor. What matters is your intention to release fully through your upper body.

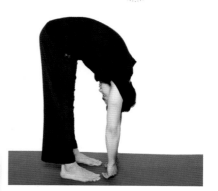

Continue to release forward, bringing your hands to the floor.

variation 1

For a variation on the stretch, interlace your fingers and place your hands at the base of your skull. Allow the extra weight to gently deepen your forward fold.

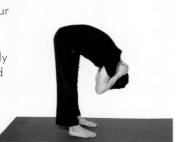

keeping it easy

You may choose to practice Standing Forward Fold with your knees bent. This is particularly wonderful to try if you have any discomfort in your lower back.

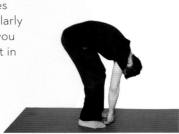

variation 2

You can also interlace your hands behind your back, and ...

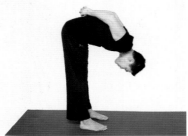

... when folding forward allow your arms to drop toward and over your head as far as they will go.

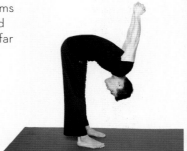

release   To release, slowly roll up to standing, imagining you are stacking bone on top of bone as you do. End in Mountain Pose.

Reclining Knee to Shoulder

Reclining Knee to Shoulder provides a rotation throughout the whole spine. Moving with breath, this is a wonderful way to release strain and tension from the back. This pose also "wrings out" and cleanses the organs of the abdomen.

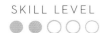
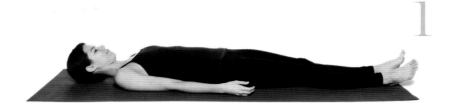

1 Lie flat on the mat, hands to your sides. Breathe deep into your belly, feeling your whole body fill with breath.

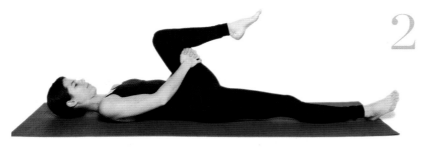

2 Using both hands, pick up your left leg from under your thigh.

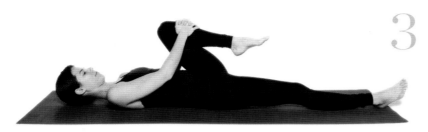

3   Inhale, then exhale, pulling your knee in toward your chest.

Keep both shoulders flat on the mat.

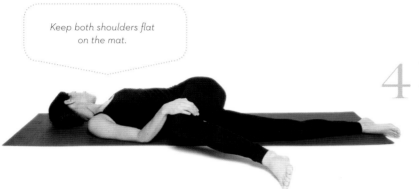

4   Using your right hand, gently bring your left knee across your body. Extend your left arm out to the left side, hand at shoulder-level.

Gaze toward your left fingertips. You can also close your eyes in this posture, feeling the shape from the inside-out.

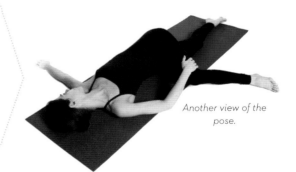

Another view of the pose.

keep it easy

With time you will stretch deeper, but don't worry about how far down your knee goes. It is more important to twist, keeping your shoulders on the earth, than to reach your knee to the mat! With each exhale, imagine your body melting into this shape further.

release

To release, inhale, then exhale, unwinding your lower body to bring your knee back to center. From there, lie on the mat with your neck straight, gazing upward once again. Then, do the other side!

Reclining Four

SKILL LEVEL
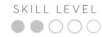

Reclining Four Pose is a wonderful and safe way to stretch all the muscles on the outside of the hip joint and release the lower back. It is often presented as an alternative to Pigeon Pose for those who want the hip stretch but find Pigeon to be too intense or painful. In this pose, your legs will make the shape of a number four.

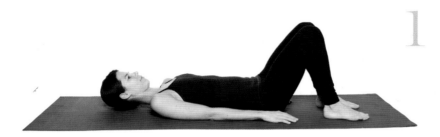

1 Lie on your back, knees bent, soles of your feet on the floor, hands at your sides.

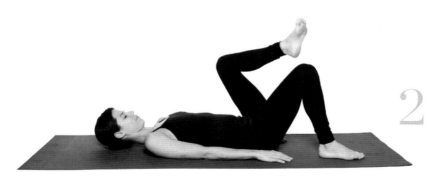

2 Bring your left leg up.

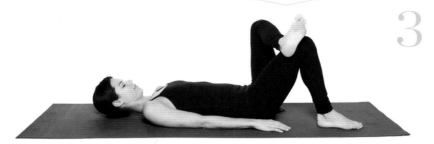

Be sure to flex through the foot.

3 Place your leg (just above your left ankle) on your right thigh, left knee facing out.

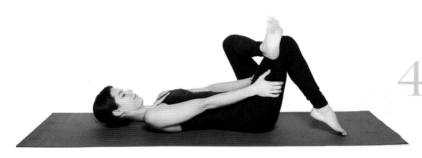

4 Bring your right leg off the floor by grabbing your right thigh.

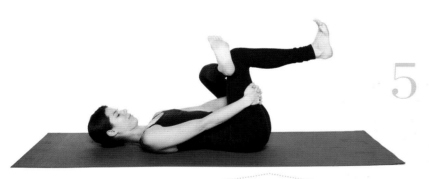

5 Inhale, then exhale, pulling your right thigh in, feeling a stretch on the outside of the hip.

You can dial up the intensity by pulling your hip closer on each exhale, or keep things more relaxed by more loosely holding your leg.

release   To release, simply rewind the steps, coming back to lying on your back, soles of your feet on the earth. Be sure to do your other leg.

Reclining Butterfly

Reclining Butterfly provides us with an opportunity to stretch the lower back, inner thighs, groin, and abdomen. This can be a wonderful pose to do toward the end of practice to release any remaining strain and stress. It's also a great shape to take some very big breaths in, given the extra space in the lungs and belly. Move carefully or skip if you have any knee injury.

SKILL LEVEL
●●○○○

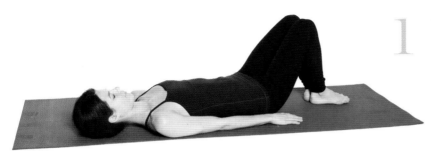

1 Lie flat on the mat, hands to your sides, palms down.

You can rock back and forth to massage your lower back.

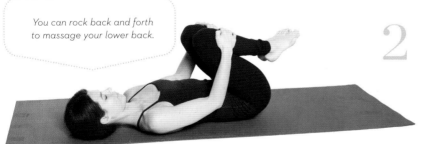

2 Bring both legs into your chest. Use your hands on your shins to support your legs.

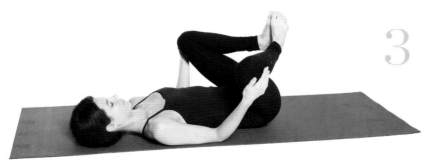

3 Put the soles of your feet together and let your legs fall open.

keep it easy

Instead of grabbing your feet, hold onto your shins.

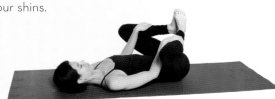

Use a strap to hold onto your feet. Gently pull your feet toward your torso.

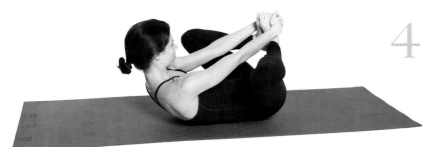

4 Reach up and grab hold of your feet from the outside edges.

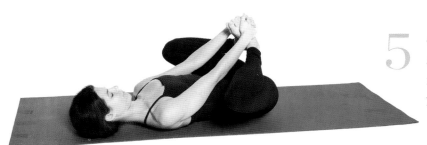

5 Continue to hold onto your feet and bring your back down to the mat. Gently pull your feet toward your seat.

release   To release, simply release the grip on your feet. Let the soles of your feet rest on the mat. Then come to lie flat on the mat.

Reclining Goddess

SKILL LEVEL
●●○○○

Reclining Goddess Pose (*Supta Baddha Konasana*) gently opens up the hips, the biggest joints in our body. If you have time, stay in this pose for several minutes, allowing the chest and hips to truly open.

1 Begin by lying flat on the floor, palms facing down.

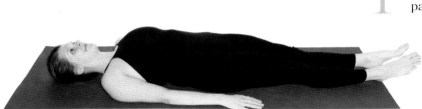

2 Bend your knees, bringing the soles of your feet to the earth.

For reclining and restorative poses such as Reclining Goddess, it's nice to bring your gaze inward. To do this, simply close your eyes. Try to bring your focus on your breath and sensations in the body, all things that are happening right now. If a thought arises, redirect your focus back to your breath.

keep it easy

For extra support, place blocks under your knees.

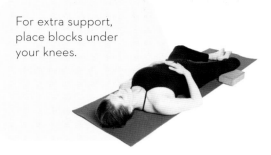

3 Bring the soles of your feet to touch each other. Let your knees flop open.

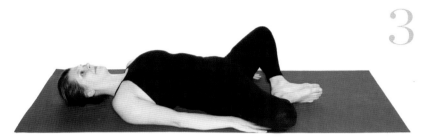

If comfortable, close your eyes.

4 Place your left hand on your belly, your right hand on your heart. Breathe into both places.

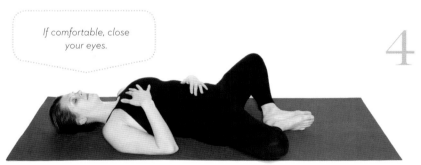

release To release, bring the palms of your hands to the outside of your knees. Slowly lift your knees upward, bringing the soles of your feet to the mat. It can be nice to allow your feet to splay wide and windshield-wiper your knees here. You can also pull your knees to your heart to massage your lower back.

restorative   141

Bridge

Bridge Pose (*Setu Bandha Sarvangasana*) stretches the chest, neck, and spine. It is known as a heart-opener for stretching the whole front body. Bridge calms the mind and provides gentle energy. It also strengthens and rejuvenates tired legs. Because the heart is elevated above the head in this pose, it is considered a gentle inversion.

SKILL LEVEL

● ● ● ○ ○

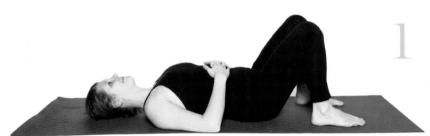

1 Lie flat on the floor with the soles of your feet on the mat, knees pointing up, and hands on your belly.

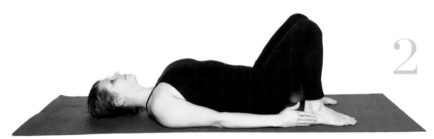

2 Draw your heels in toward your seat. Reach down and try to brush your fingertips against your heels.

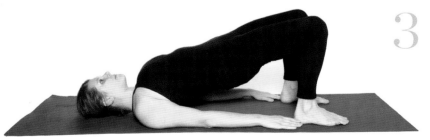

3 Take a full breath, and on the exhale push your torso up toward the ceiling.

For support, put a block under your lower back. Let your arms rest out to the sides of your body and breathe easy.

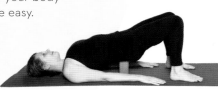

To protect your neck, be sure to keep it straight.

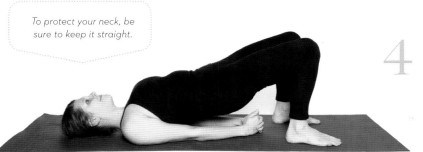

4 Interlock your fingers under your body and press into the earth with your arms and the heels of your feet.

It's normal to feel compression in your neck. In fact, this gentle compression massages the thyroid gland. Keep gazing upward to protect your neck.

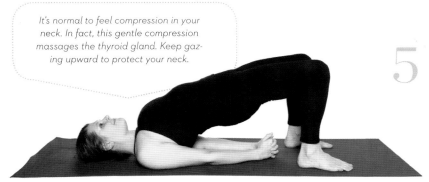

5 Press your hips to the ceiling.

Once you roll out of the shape, it's often nice to stay in the start position, with knees bent, soles of your feet on the floor. From here, gently shift your knees back and forth to massage and release your lower back. You can imagine your knees moving like windshield wipers on a car.

release

To release, remove your arms from under your body, then roll your upper, middle, then lower back to the earth.

Reclining Eagle Twist

Reclining Eagle Twist provides a full body twist, from feet through the hips and spine and the neck. We'll utilize the legs we know from Eagle Pose to intensify the stretch and rotation through the lower body. If you have any sensitivity in the knees or lower back, you can also do this twist with knees simply pressing side by side.

SKILL LEVEL

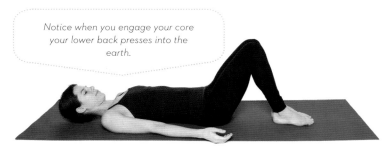

Notice when you engage your core your lower back presses into the earth.

1   Lie down on your back, feet flat on the floor. Take a few deep breaths into your belly.

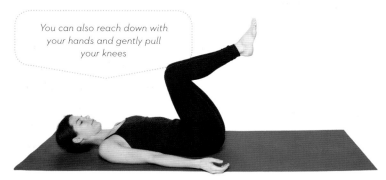

You can also reach down with your hands and gently pull your knees

2   Keeping your knees together, bring them up so your calves are parallel to the floor.

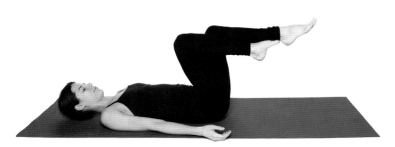

3   Cross your left leg over your right leg. This is a single twist and a fine place to stop. For a double twist, try tucking your left foot behind your right calf.

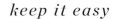

Instead of intertwining
your legs, just keep them
together and bring them
over to the side.

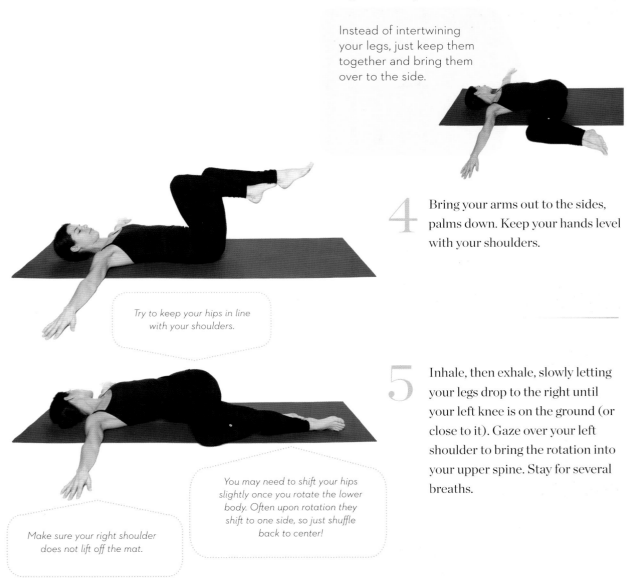

4 Bring your arms out to the sides,
palms down. Keep your hands level
with your shoulders.

*Try to keep your hips in line
with your shoulders.*

5 Inhale, then exhale, slowly letting
your legs drop to the right until
your left knee is on the ground (or
close to it). Gaze over your left
shoulder to bring the rotation into
your upper spine. Stay for several
breaths.

*You may need to shift your hips
slightly once you rotate the lower
body. Often upon rotation they
shift to one side, so just shuffle
back to center!*

*Make sure your right shoulder
does not lift off the mat.*

release   To release, inhale then exhale your lower body back to center. From there, unwind your
legs, then try winding them to the other side. Bring your knees to the opposite side,
then shift your head to the opposite direction, as well. Once both sides are done, bring
your legs back to center, then rock up to sit.

GOING

DEEPER

Unless you try to do something

beyond what you have already

mastered, you will never grow.

-Ralph Waldo Emerson

ADVANCED VARIATIONS

Once you feel comfortable in the poses in Part 2, you can try taking things a bit further. In this section, you'll find variations of poses you already know. Here you can stretch further, move deeper, and test your mental and emotional balance and flexibility. This is all about building on what we've already learned.

Use your breath as a guide. If your breath becomes labored, you may want to ease up and back out of the shape a bit. Aim to keep your breath even and full in all of these advanced variations. Remember, it is the deep full breathing (try your *ujjayi*!) that adds magic to the poses, helping us to link the body and the mind.

With time and patience, you'll find you can go further than you ever thought you could.

Seated Wide Leg Straddle

SKILL LEVEL
●○○○○

We can take our Seated Wide Leg Straddle further by adding in a forward bend. This will give a deeper stretch in the spine, legs, hips, and groin.

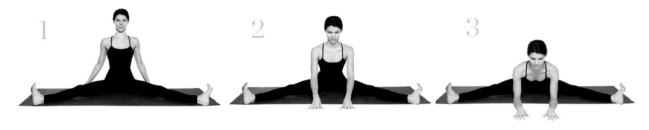

1 2 3

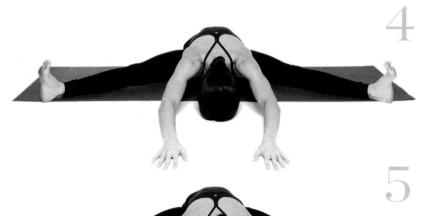

4 Extend your arms fully, palms down, bringing your head as close to the earth as possible.

5 Continue to let your head drop. Reach for your feet, grabbing hold of the inside of the soles.

Gaze down or close your eyes. Focus on how you feel here, not what you see. Feel the sensations of this deep stretch and breathe!

No matter how far forward you can reach, breathe fully. With time your muscles will release further, providing a deeper and deeper stretch. But enjoy where you are!

Low Squat

Our Low Squat becomes more advanced by adding a side stretch and heart opener.

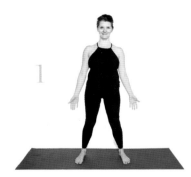

1

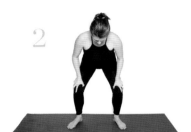

2

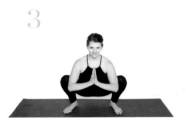

3

Feel the expansion in this shape even though you are low to the ground and in a small shape. With each exhale feel your palm planted into the earth and with each inhale feel the openness of the heart toward the sky.

4   Straighten out your left arm and place your hand on the ground. Stretch your right arm up to the sky, looking up at your right fingertips.

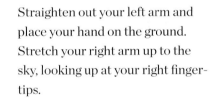

advanced variations   151

Fire Log

Fire Log Pose becomes more advanced when we add a forward fold. Here, we pursue a deep stretch in the hips and in the back of the body. Stay for several minutes—or deep breaths—to allow the hips to release.

SKILL LEVEL

●●○○○

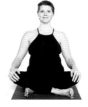 1

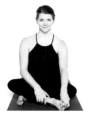 2

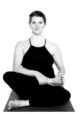 3

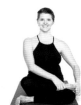 4

5

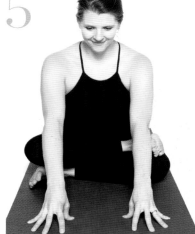

Begin to walk your fingertips forward, leading with the heart. Think of reaching out, then down.

6

As you let your head drop, let your gaze drop also.

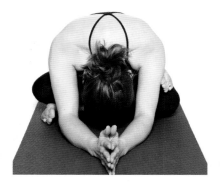

Bring your hands into prayer pose and let your upper body melt down toward your legs and the mat.

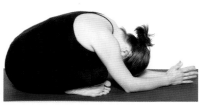

Side shot of the pose, head down.

Butterfly Pose becomes more advanced by adding a forward fold into the mix. Here we stretch the back of the body and melt toward the earth. Hold for several breaths to really release and stretch.

Butterfly

SKILL LEVEL
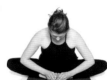

1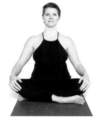

2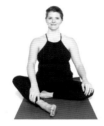

3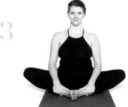

4

5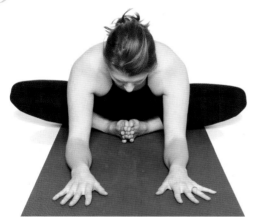

6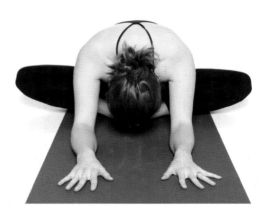

Walk your fingers out in front, leading with the heart. Place your elbows and forearms on the mat, palms down.

Inhale, then exhale and sink into the pose, letting your head release. Close your eyes and breathe.

advanced variations

High Lunge Twist

High Lunge Twist provides a chance to develop balance, concentration, and lower body strength while twisting the spine and abdominal organs. Twisting through the spine promotes spine health, and the spine is the central energy channel of the body. Be sure to do both sides!

SKILL LEVEL
●●●○○

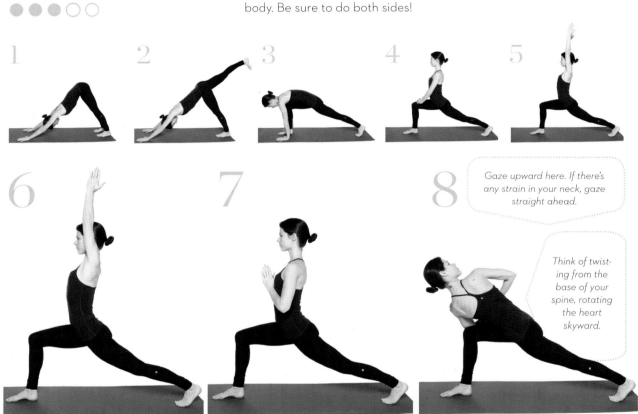

Gaze upward here. If there's any strain in your neck, gaze straight ahead.

Think of twisting from the base of your spine, rotating the heart skyward.

Press your palms together overhead. Aim to keep your shoulders away from your ears even though your palms are pressed.

Inhale, then exhale, bringing your hands down in front of your heart. Balance here for a few breaths. On the inhale, feel the heart rise into the prayer hands. On the exhale, sink a bit lower into the 90 degree angle of your front leg.

Inhale, then exhale, bringing your left elbow to the outside edge of your right knee. See if you can use the leverage of your left elbow to knee to rotate your chest up toward the sky.

Cobra

Cobra Pose can be made more advanced by deepening the backbend in the shape. By engaging the lower body as well as the upper body, we can move deeper into a back and leg stretch.

SKILL LEVEL
●●●○○

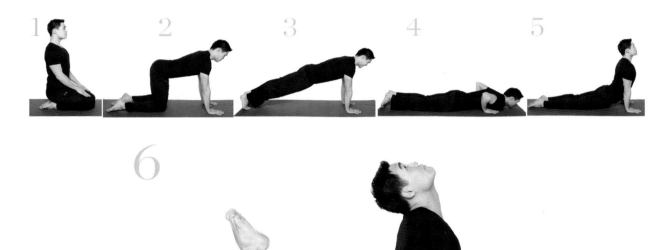

Bend your knees and bring your toes toward your head. Bring your head back and look up. Someday, with time and practice, your head may touch your feet!

Balancing Tabletop

SKILL LEVEL
● ● ○ ○ ○

We can make our Balancing Tabletop more advanced by adding a bow shape with the arm and leg. This is an added balance challenge. This pose stretches the spine and invigorates the mind.

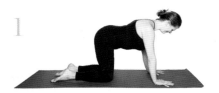 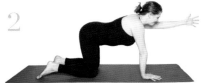 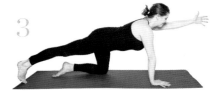

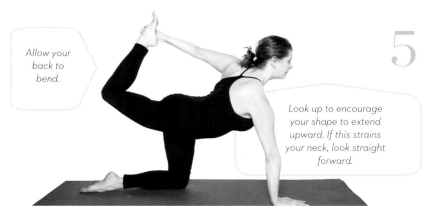

Lift your back leg so your thigh is parallel to the floor.

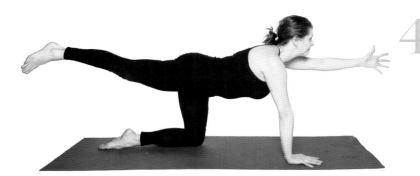

Allow your back to bend.

Look up to encourage your shape to extend upward. If this strains your neck, look straight forward.

Reach back with your extended arm and grab your foot. Press into your hand to create more opening in the heart.

Three-Legged Dog

We can add a hip opener to our Downward Facing Dog by lifting one leg at a time. This gives a stretch in the hip itself and also the side body. It also adds a balance challenge to the traditional Downward Facing Dog.

SKILL LEVEL
●●○○○

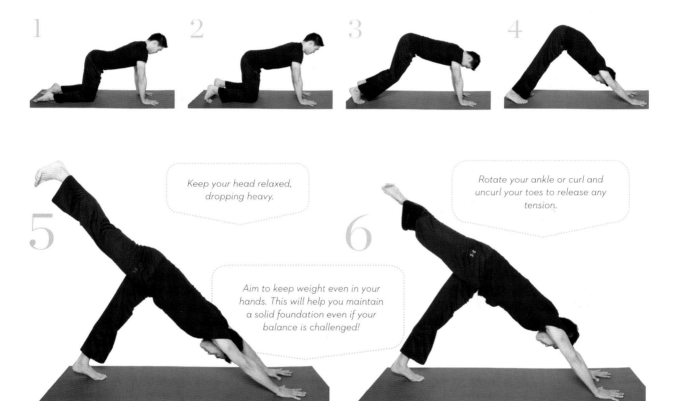

1

2

3

4

5

Keep your head relaxed, dropping heavy.

Aim to keep weight even in your hands. This will help you maintain a solid foundation even if your balance is challenged!

6

Rotate your ankle or curl and uncurl your toes to release any tension.

Inhale and bring your right leg high.

Bend your raised leg to a 90-degree angle.

advanced variations

Tree

Tree Pose becomes more challenging when we add variation to the upper body. By swaying consciously from one side to the other we move balance away from the body's center and add a side stretch. We engage new muscles and practice staying cool under the pressure of being off center.

SKILL LEVEL
●●●○○

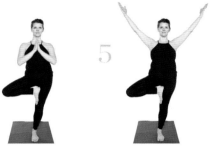

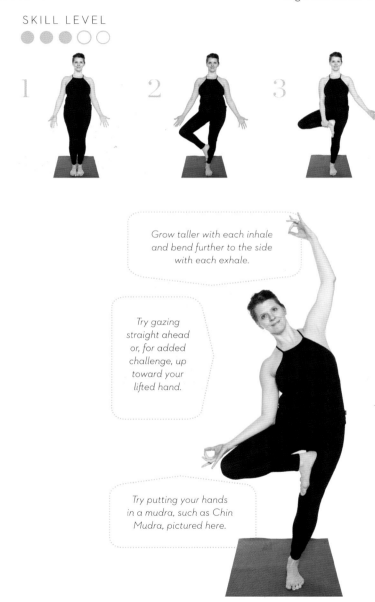

Grow taller with each inhale and bend further to the side with each exhale.

Try gazing straight ahead or, for added challenge, up toward your lifted hand.

Try putting your hands in a mudra, such as Chin Mudra, pictured here.

6 Reaching from your hips, bend to the right side, resting your lower forearm on your thigh. Reach the left arm up and slightly over the body, feeling a side stretch.

Remember, if you fall it's a wonderful opportunity to try again! If you do fall out of the shape, notice how you react and see if you can approach the challenge with play and a sense of non-attachment.

Come into a full Boat Pose to fully engage this core strengthener and the focus that comes with it!

Boat

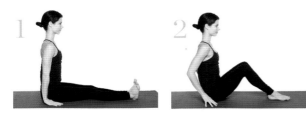

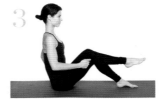

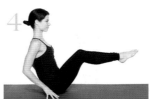

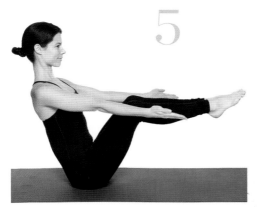

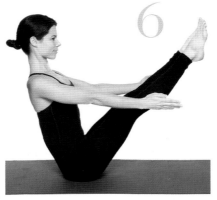

Straighten your arms out at shoulder
height, palms up. Engage your core,
thinking of pulling belly button to
spine. Keep your knees bent.

For a full Boat, straighten your legs
and turn your palms inward.

The important thing here is feeling your core engaged and
heart elevated. Choose your leg variation, bent or straight,
with that in mind. Don't compromise your straight back and
elevated heart for a certain leg shape!

Twisting Boat

Boat Pose is a wonderful core strengthener. By adding a twist, we can strengthen the side muscles of the core, which are often hard to reach.

SKILL LEVEL
● ● ● ○ ○

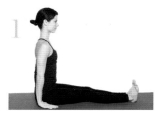 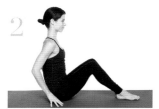 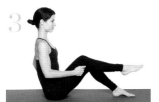 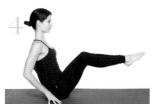

Avoid any slumping through the back!

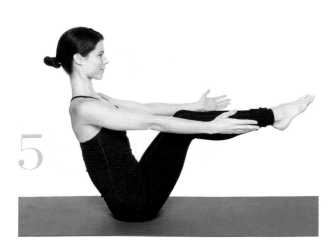

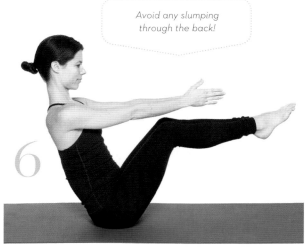

Straighten your arms at the level of your shins, palms up. Pull your belly toward your spine to engage the core muscles.

Bring your hands together, palms pressing, in front of your shins. Keep the heart lifted.

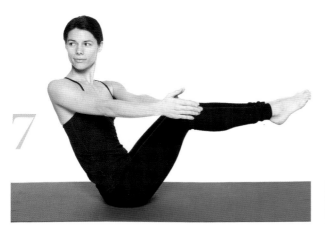

Inhale, then exhale and twist your upper body to the right, looking over your right shoulder. Inhale.

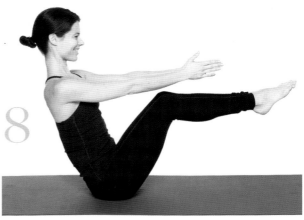

Exhale, coming back to center.

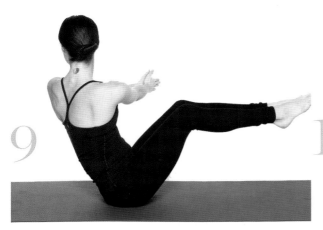

Inhale, then exhale, twisting to the left, looking over your left shoulder. Inhale.

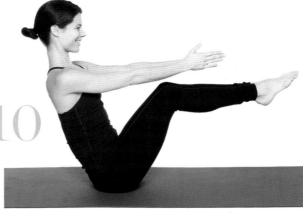

Exhale, coming back to center.

This pose is all about the breath. Move from one shape to the next on the exhale and inhale. Take note of the breath instructions and work them into your practice. These poses move in a flow, so you'll be moving with breath to "row your boat," working all the muscles in the core of your body.

Floor Bow (Superhero)

Floor Bow offers a wonderful stretch through the entire front of the body, opening the heart while strengthening the spine and legs. This pose also stimulates the abdominal organs and digestion. Avoid if you have a serious lower back injury.

SKILL LEVEL
●●●○○

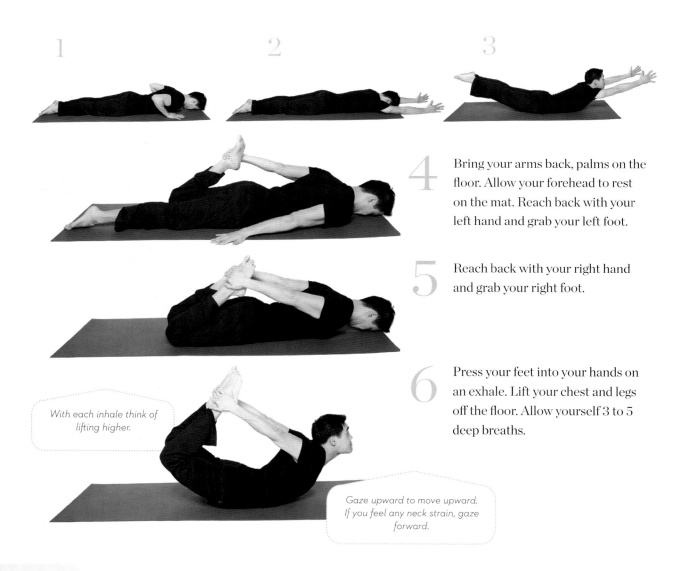

1

2

3

4 Bring your arms back, palms on the floor. Allow your forehead to rest on the mat. Reach back with your left hand and grab your left foot.

5 Reach back with your right hand and grab your right foot.

6 Press your feet into your hands on an exhale. Lift your chest and legs off the floor. Allow yourself 3 to 5 deep breaths.

With each inhale think of lifting higher.

Gaze upward to move upward. If you feel any neck strain, gaze forward.

Half Moon

We can make Half Moon Pose more advanced by adding a backbend while in the balancing shape. Here you'll feel extension through the heart and a wonderful stretch through the thigh.

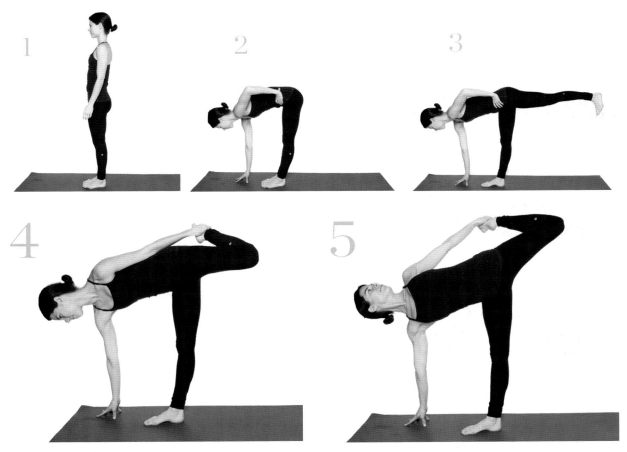

Grasp the top of your left foot with your left hand. Begin to press into your hand.

Allow your body to open to the left. Gaze upward or straight ahead. Continue to press into your hand to stretch through your thigh. Feel the lift in the heart and the bow shape in your body as you arch through your back.

Half Boat

Half Boat Pose is a wonderful core strengthener, leading to strong abs and a healthy back and spine! If you have any sensitivity in your lower back, try the variation.

SKILL LEVEL
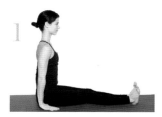

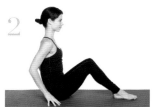 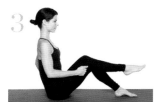 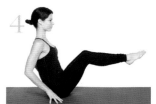

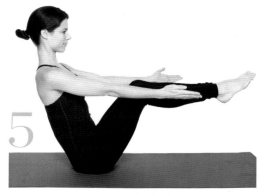

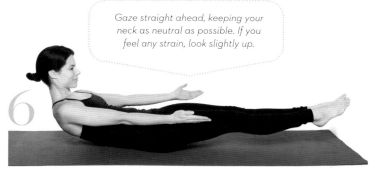

Gaze straight ahead, keeping your neck as neutral as possible. If you feel any strain, look slightly up.

Straighten and lift your arms up to the level of your shins, palms face up. Engage your core, pulling the belly button toward the spine. This is your full Boat Pose.

Inhale, then exhale, straightening your legs and lowering your upper body at the same time. Use your stomach muscles to lower only half way down, keeping your shoulders and legs off the floor.

keep it easy

If you feel any strain at all, tent your fingers by your hips for extra support.

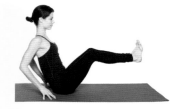

Tiptoe Squat

We can make Tiptoe Squat more advanced by adding to the balance challenge and lifting a leg. This pose cultivates patience along with balance, and strengthens core and leg muscles while stretching the foot and ankle deeply.

SKILL LEVEL
● ● ● ● ○

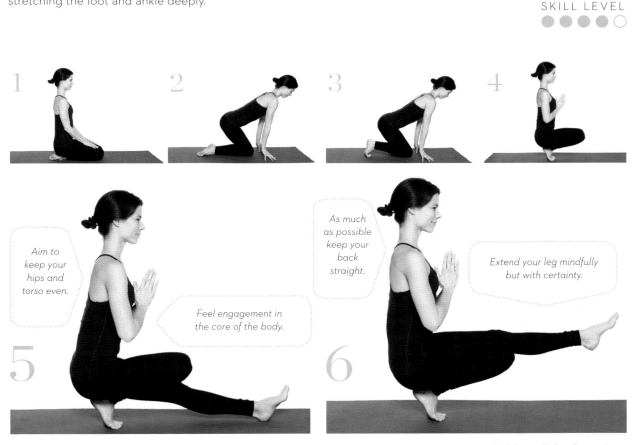

Aim to keep your hips and torso even.

Feel engagement in the core of the body.

As much as possible keep your back straight.

Extend your leg mindfully but with certainty.

On an exhale, straighten your left leg, resting your heel on the floor.

Again on an exhale, raise your left leg off the floor. Aim to make your left thigh parallel to your right.

This is a tricky balance challenge. It is normal to fall out of the shape! Simply get right back into it if you do. The floor is not far from you if you fall.

To achieve this balancing shape you must have a "go for it!" attitude. Hesitation won't help you here. Confidence will aid you.

advanced variations   165

Fish

Add a core strengthening challenge to the regular heart and throat opening Fish Pose provides. Here the leg lift will work muscles deep in the lower abdomen. Avoid or vary this modification if you have a lower back or neck injury or pain.

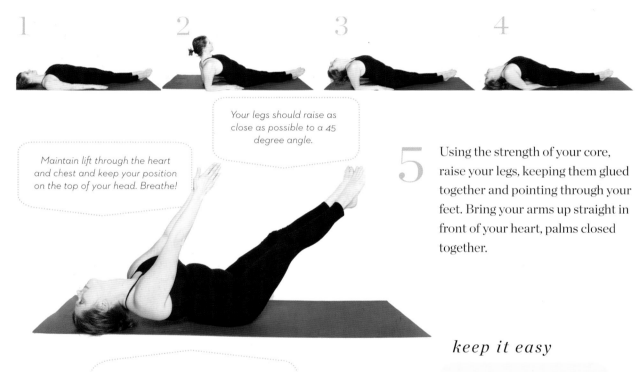

1 2 3 4

Your legs should raise as close as possible to a 45 degree angle.

Maintain lift through the heart and chest and keep your position on the top of your head. Breathe!

5 Using the strength of your core, raise your legs, keeping them glued together and pointing through your feet. Bring your arms up straight in front of your heart, palms closed together.

Remember to engage your core in this posture! The center of your body will help keep your fish tail strong and long.

keep it easy

If anything becomes strained or uncomfortable, mindfully lower your legs and arms coming to lie on your back. From here, you can transition back into your regular Fish Pose.

Revolved Triangle

Triangle Pose becomes Revolved Triangle simply by changing the position of the hands and rotating the torso in the opposite direction from the regular Triangle motion.

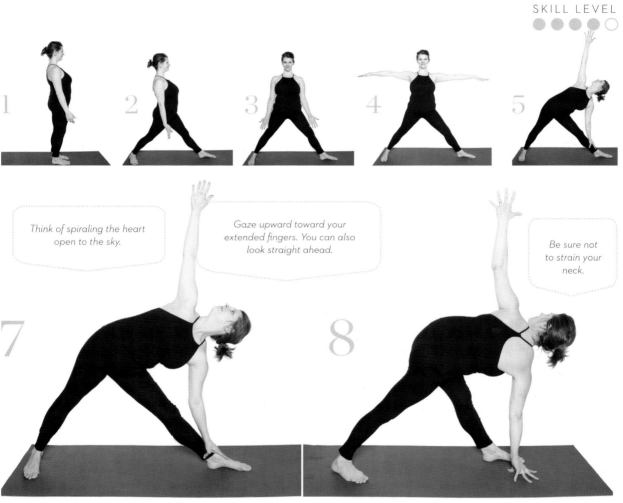

1 2 3 4 5

Think of spiraling the heart open to the sky.

Gaze upward toward your extended fingers. You can also look straight ahead.

Be sure not to strain your neck.

7

Bring your left hand all way down to the top of your foot.

8

Bring your top arm down to the floor, fingers tented. Rotate toward your front leg and raise your other arm up.

advanced variations   167

Cow Face

We can make Cow Face Pose more advanced by adding a forward-fold into the mix.

SKILL LEVEL
●●●●○

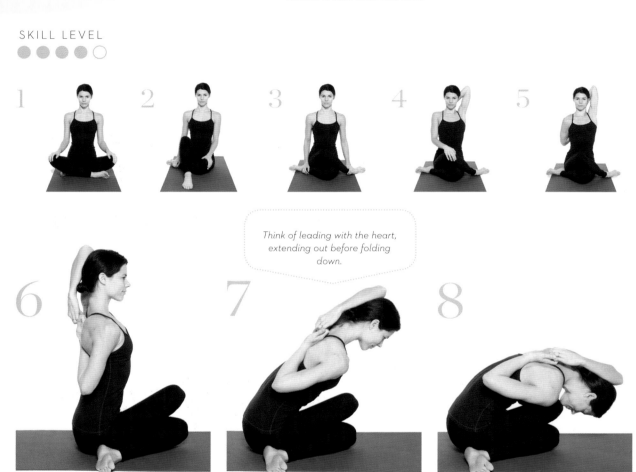

Think of leading with the heart, extending out before folding down.

Sit upright with hands clasped.

Inhale, then exhale, gently bending forward at the hips.

Release your head completely. It may touch your knee or it may simply drop, but aim to release any neck tension.

Revolved Half Moon

Revolved Half Moon provides a balance challenge and a twist throughout the spine at the same time. This pose strengthens and tones the standing leg, massages the organs of the belly from the inside out, and promotes spine health. It also develops mental focus and concentration.

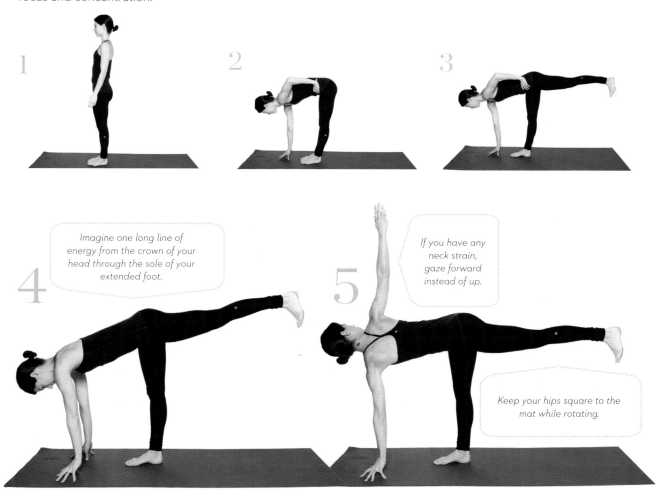

1

2

3

4

Imagine one long line of energy from the crown of your head through the sole of your extended foot.

5

If you have any neck strain, gaze forward instead of up.

Keep your hips square to the mat while rotating.

Reach the fingertips of both hands to the mat. Square your shoulders and hips to the earth. Gaze down.

Extend your right arm to the sky, looking up at your fingers. Open the heart to the sky.

Pigeon (Forward)

We can make Pigeon Pose more advanced by adding a forward fold that deepens the stretch through the hip and is nice to stay in for several breaths (or even minutes).

SKILL LEVEL
● ● ● ● ○

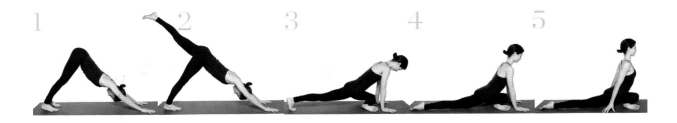

Keep your elbows shoulder-width apart.

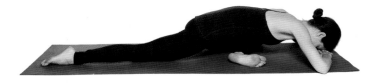

6 Walk your fingertips forward and place your forearms on the ground, palms down.

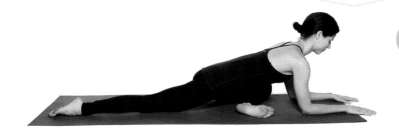

7 Make a pillow out of your hands. Allow your forehead to rest on your forearms. Stay here for several minutes if possible, allowing the large hip joint to release.

Pigeon (Back)

We can also advance Pigeon Pose by adding a backbend, allowing for a lift through the heart and stretch in the thigh. Start with steps 1-5 on the previous page.

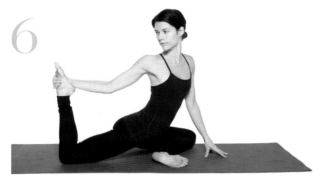

Bend your right knee and bring the leg up. Reach back with your right arm and grasp your foot. Keep your hips square to the mat. This is a fine place to stop.

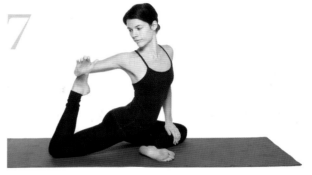

If you like, try bringing your foot into the crook of your arm.

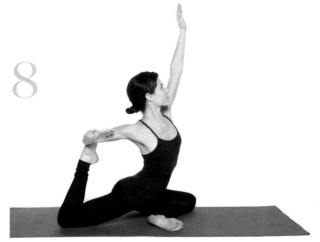

Reach up to the sky with your left arm, looking forward.

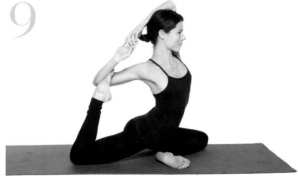

Bend both arms and try to hold hands with yourself. Keep your shoulders square to the front of the mat and gaze ahead. You can also use a strap or grab ahold of your shirt.

advanced variations 171

Extended Side Angle

Some small changes in the upper body can make Extended Side Angle more advanced.

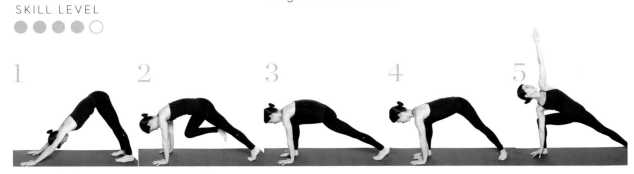

1   2   3   4   5

If there's ever any neck strain when looking upward, simply look straight ahead.

Imagine you are shining your heart toward the sky, spiraling from the base of your spine.

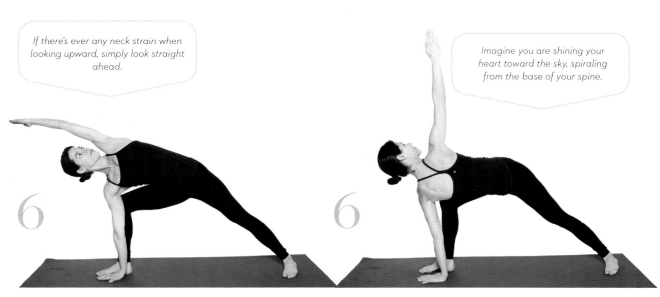

6   6

Variation 1: Extend your left arm overhead so the arm reaches over your ear. Gaze upward or straight ahead.

Variation 2: To create Revolved Side Angle, place your left hand on the ground to the inside of your right foot. Reach your right arm up to the sky and follow the arm with your gaze, looking up.

Eagle

To make Eagle Pose more challenging we'll add a forward fold
into the mix. Here we begin to bow our heads to our hearts,
extending through the back and hips.

1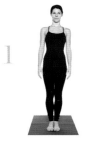

2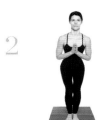

3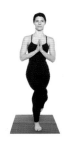

4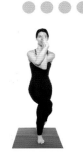

5

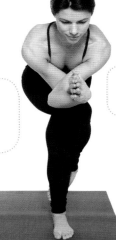

Make sure your knees are still aligned over your ankles. If they extend beyond your ankles you could harm the knee joints.

Think of reaching forward, then down.

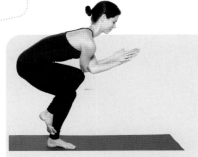

Side angle of final pose.

Bend forward from the hips, leading with the heart.
See if you can bring your elbows to your knees or even
beyond your knees.

advanced variations   173

Side Plank 1

Our Side Plank becomes more advanced by adding some variation in the leg position and further challenging balance. You will strengthen your core all around the torso as well as arms and legs in this active shape.

SKILL LEVEL
●●●●○

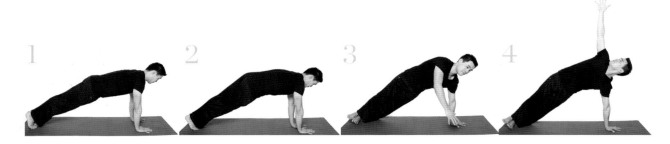

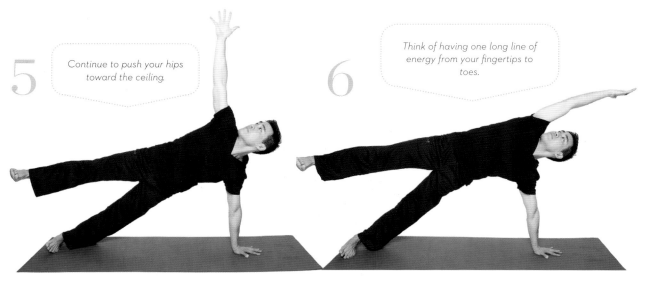

5
Continue to push your hips toward the ceiling.

6
Think of having one long line of energy from your fingertips to toes.

On an exhale, lift your top leg away from your bottom leg. Flex through your foot.

Reach your arm overhead.

Side Plank 2

As you become comfortable with Side Plank you can begin to
have fun with variations of the upper leg, such as adding Tree
Pose to our Side Plank for a balance challenge.

1 2 3 4

5

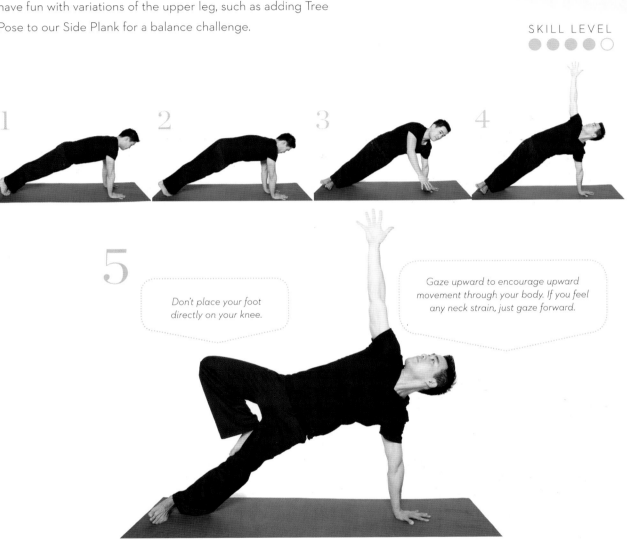

*Don't place your foot
directly on your knee.*

*Gaze upward to encourage upward
movement through your body. If you feel
any neck strain, just gaze forward.*

Try coming into a Tree Pose in your legs while in Side Plank. Place
your right foot on your left leg, above or below the knee. Raise your
hand upward, fingers extended.

Reclining Hero

We can add extra challenge to our Reclining Hero by deepening our recline. Here the upper body will take on a shape similar to that of Fish Pose, opening the throat and stretching the chest. Move to your own level of comfort; skip this variation if you have a neck injury.

SKILL LEVEL

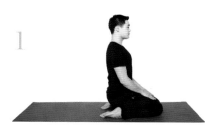

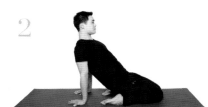

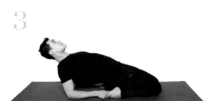

4

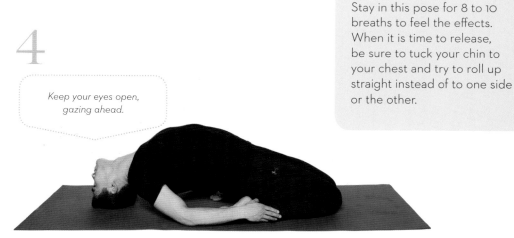

Keep your eyes open, gazing ahead.

Stay in this pose for 8 to 10 breaths to feel the effects. When it is time to release, be sure to tuck your chin to your chest and try to roll up straight instead of to one side or the other.

On an exhale, bring the top of your head to the mat while your hands grab onto your feet. Feel the stretch through your throat, the openness in the front body.

Dolphin

Dolphin Pose can be made more advanced by adding movement to the shape. Here we will "swim" the shape forward and back, building more strength in the shoulders, upper back, and legs.

SKILL LEVEL
● ● ● ● ●

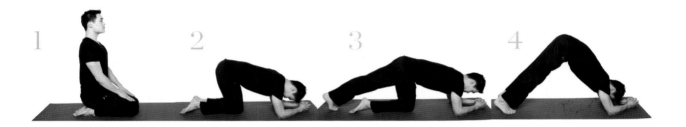

1   2   3   4

5

Keep your core engaged as you move.

As you shift your weight forward, continue to push your forearms into the floor, moving your shoulders away from your ears as you do. Aim not to dump weight in the shoulders, but rather lift out of them.

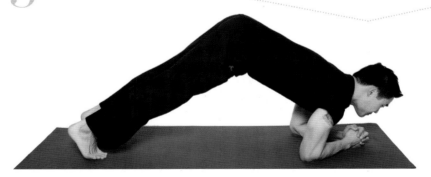

Inhale, then exhale while shifting weight forward, aiming to bring your chin over your hands. Gaze slightly forward. Inhale there, then exhale, coming back to the original pose. Repeat, moving forward and back on inhales and exhales.

The best way to overcome fear

is to face with equanimity the

situation of which one is afraid.

—B.K.S. Iyengar

ADVANCED POSES

Once you feel comfortable with the poses outlined in Part 2, give these advanced poses a try. In these shapes, you'll be called to try things like balancing on your hands or head, and moving into deep backbends or twists. Aim to move smoothly, keeping your breath even. The most advanced thing you can do is cultivate the quality of paying attention inside these shapes.

Advanced postures give us an opportunity to practice staying calm even when things get tricky. Notice your thoughts, how your breath reacts, and what emotions arise when you face a challenge like Headstand. Try to notice without judgment, only curiosity. From there, you begin to learn about yourself and know when you can push yourself further and when to rest. These poses are also a chance to practice patience, build confidence, and to have fun.

Camel

Camel Pose (*Ustrasana*) is a deep backbend and heart-opener. In this way, it stretches the whole front of the body, from ankles to thighs to chest to throat. It is a wonderful counter-stretch for those who work slightly hunched at computers for most of the day. Proceed gently or avoid if you have a serious lower back injury or high blood pressure.

SKILL LEVEL
●●●●○

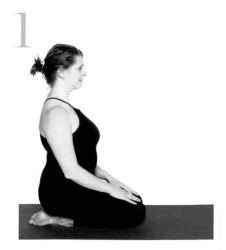

1

Begin in Hero's Pose, sitting with hips to heels, palms resting on your thighs.

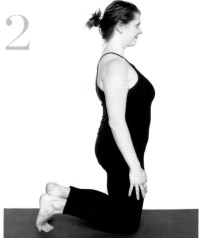

2

Come to standing on your knees, tucking your toes under.

The space between your knees should be the width of both your fists placed together. This is hip-width.

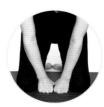

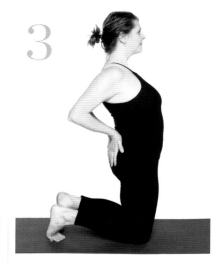

3

Place your hands on your lower back, fingers pointing down.

You may feel lightheaded or dizzy in this shape. Again, this is often because we keep this part of the body protected and more closed. Try to breathe through sensations, but if they become too strong, come to sit in Hero's Pose.

Because we experience many emotions in the heart center, and often keep it protected with our shoulders slightly hunched, this great opening can release a flood of emotions. Just remember to breathe, know that it's positive to release feelings no matter what they are attached to, and know that all things do pass. This effect can be part of Camel Pose's power.

keep it easy

If you experience sensitivity or pain in your knees, place a folded mat or blanket under them.

4

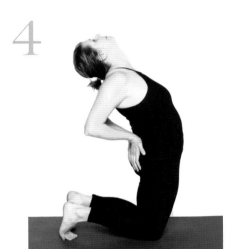

5

Gaze straight back in this pose. Keep your eyes open.

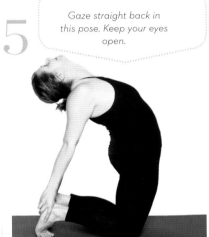

take it a step further

For more of a stretch, untuck your toes so the tops of your feet rest on the mat.

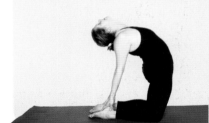

Begin to bend back, opening your heart and throat. Allow your head to gently drop. If you are a beginner you can stop here.

Walk your fingers down and grab onto your heels. Let your head drop back. Open up your heart and gently push your hips forward with each exhale.

release Do your best to raise up out of the pose by moving straight up, both hips coming up at once, to avoid straining the lower back. Bring your hands to your lower back, inhale, then exhale raising forward. Then come to sit in Hero's Pose.

Bow

In Bow Pose (*Dhanurasana*) the legs and torso represent the body of a bow, and the arms represent the string. Bow Pose stretches the front of the body, from the ankles through the hip flexors right up to the abdomen, chest, and throat. Lying on the belly in this way stimulates the organs of the abdomen. Avoid if you have a serious lower back injury or high blood pressure.

SKILL LEVEL
● ● ● ● ○

1 Begin by lying face-down, hands at your sides with palms down and forehead on the mat.

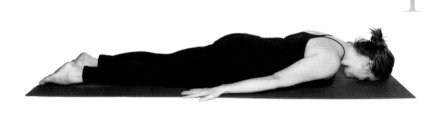

2 Reach back with your left hand and capture your left ankle, bringing it to your buttocks.

You may find yourself naturally rocking with the breath as you inhale and exhale. Keep the breath full and the gaze soft but intent, and enjoy the ride.

If you can't grab your ankles, hold onto your pant leg instead. Either way, lift your knees and chest.

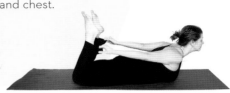

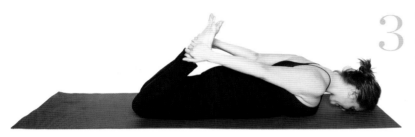

3 With your right hand, reach back and grab your right ankle and draw it in toward your buttocks.

Avoid looking down in this pose. If you have any neck strain keep the gaze more forward than up.

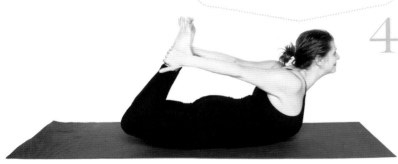

4 Pressing the feet into the hands, lift your knees and chest up, looking forward and a little up.

release   Release the pose on an exhale, letting go of your feet and slowly lowering your legs and chest to the earth. Lying on your belly, turn your head to the right, allowing the left ear to rest on the mat.

Thunderbolt Twist

SKILL LEVEL
●●●●○

Thunderbolt Twist strengthens the ankles and legs while stretching and rotating the spine. This pose also "wrings out" the organs of the abdomen, helping with digestion.

> If you can't rotate your thumbs to reach heart center right away, don't be discouraged. It takes a lot of flexibility.

1

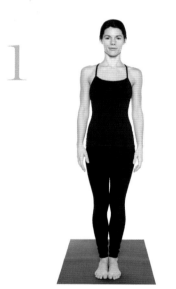

Begin in Mountain Pose, arms at your sides

2

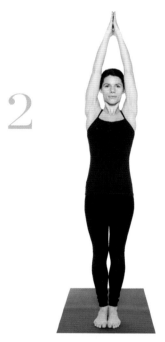

Bring your arms above your head, palms pressed together in a prayer shape.

3

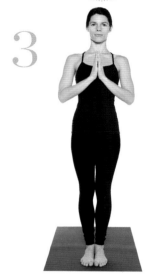

Inhale, then exhale, bringing your hands down to heart center.

If your prayer hands reach heart center, you can try extending both arms open in a Fly Away shape, feeling a full wingspan.

Be sure your knees are still over your ankles to protect the knee joints. To ensure weight is in the heels, try wiggling the toes and then placing them back down to the mat.

Press your elbow into your leg as leverage to twist open and upward. With each inhale, twist open even more. With each exhale, sink deeper into your chair shape, being sure your knees stay aligned over your ankles.

4

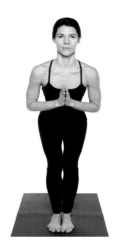

5

Gaze upward.

Often in this shape, one knee wants to pop forward in front of the other. Try to keep your knees in line as you twist open and up.

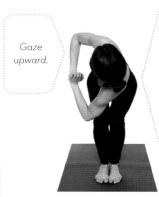

Slowly sit back and down, making sure your weight is in your heels.

Inhale, then exhale, twisting from the base of your spine toward the left. Place your left elbow outside your right leg above the knee.

release To release, bring your hands and your torso back to center, facing forward. On an inhale, stand up to Mountain Pose.

Plow

Plow Pose (*Halasana*) is a powerful shape that calms the mind, stretches the shoulders and spine, and stimulates the thyroid gland and digestive organs. Avoid or proceed carefully if you have a neck injury. If you are menstruating, pay attention to your body to see if this inversion and compression is right for you.

SKILL LEVEL

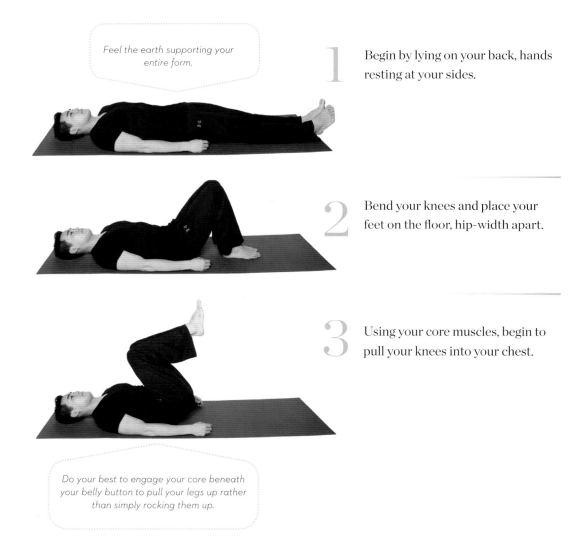

Feel the earth supporting your entire form.

1 Begin by lying on your back, hands resting at your sides.

2 Bend your knees and place your feet on the floor, hip-width apart.

3 Using your core muscles, begin to pull your knees into your chest.

Do your best to engage your core beneath your belly button to pull your legs up rather than simply rocking them up.

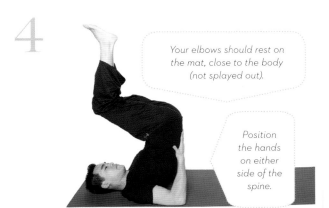

4

Your elbows should rest on the mat, close to the body (not splayed out).

Position the hands on either side of the spine.

Place your hands on your lower back with fingers pointing upward toward your feet. Begin to extend your legs.

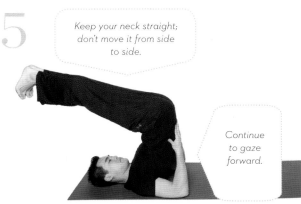

5

Keep your neck straight; don't move it from side to side.

Continue to gaze forward.

Allow your legs to shift over your head. You will feel a gentle compression in your neck. Flex your feet.

6

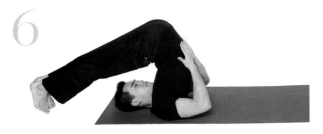

Bring your legs all the way overhead and see if your toes can touch the floor above your crown. Stay in this pose for 8 to 10 deep breaths.

keep it easy

For added support, use a chair in Plow Pose. Place your legs on the chair instead of reaching them all the way to the earth. Continue to keep your hands on your lower back and your neck straight. Flex your feet.

variation

Try to place your hands palms down, arms shoulder-width apart. Press into the earth with your hands and continue to move the legs toward the mat, or touch the mat with your feet.

Another variation is Deaf Man's Pose. Here you will bend your knees and bring them to either side of your ears. Often this shape can relieve tension in the lower back.

release Exhale, using your core to slowly lower your legs back overhead and to the mat, coming to lie down flat. Take your time; avoid the temptation to fling yourself out of the shape. Use mindfulness and muscle to lower slowly.

Shoulder Stand

Shoulder Stand (*Sarvangasana*) is a wonderful, safe, powerful inversion. It is often nicknamed the "Queen" of poses for its many benefits. Shoulder Stand increases metabolism, soothes the nervous system, and reverses the flow of gravity, revitalizing the entire body. Avoid or proceed carefully if you have a shoulder or neck injury. Many women avoid inversions such as Shoulder Stand while menstruating, especially during the first three days of the cycle, but listen to your body.

SKILL LEVEL
●●●●○

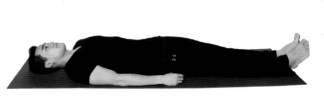

1 Begin by lying on your back, hands resting at your sides.

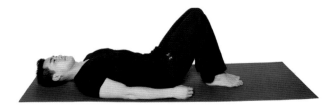

2 Bend your knees and place your feet on the floor, shoulder-width apart.

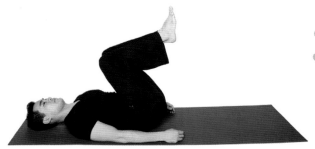

3 Using your core, begin to draw your knees into your chest.

4

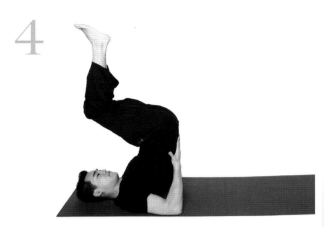

5

Align your heels over your shoulders.

Keep your neck in position; don't move it from side to side.

Place your hands on your lower back for support, fingers pointing toward your toes. Begin to extend your legs.

Extend your legs straight, keeping your legs together. Either flex or point the feet, then engage the feet to keep energy there.

keep it easy

To avoid dumping weight in the shoulders think of extending the toes further toward the sky with each inhale. Press into the earth with your shoulders and elbows, reaching your toes up. Keep your feet engaged. It's all about extending up!

Some yogis like to place a folded blanket under the shoulders and upper back for extra cushion and for extra space for the neck. Fold a blanket into a thin rectangle. Place the blanket so your shoulders and upper back are on the blanket but your neck and head will be off the blanket. From here, come into the pose as normal. This variation sometimes helps if you feel too much strain through the neck in Shoulder Stand.

release To release, roll out slowly, using your core muscles to lower your legs. It can be nice to pass through Plow Pose on the way to the earth. Come to lie on the mat and either rest here, feeling the effects of Shoulder Stand, or come into Fish Pose to reverse the direction of compression in the throat.

Crow

Crow Pose (*Bakasana*) is an arm balancing pose. Learning this pose can create a surge of self-confidence and a feeling of almost flying, like a crow. This pose also improves overall balance while strengthening the arms, shoulders, and core (it takes core strength to lift up!). This is a safe, fun arm balance to try as a beginner since, if you fall, the floor is not far away.

SKILL LEVEL
●●●●○

1

Try to keep your back straight and heart lifted.

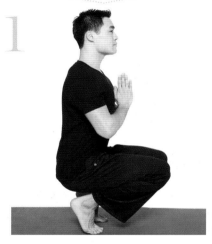

Begin in Tiptoe Squat, balancing on flexed toes. Place your hands together in front of your heart. Inhale.

2

Your knees should flare out. This alone provides a stretch through the groin and hips.

Your elbows should be like small shelves.

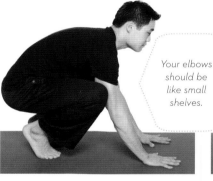

Exhale, bringing your hands down to the mat, palms flat on the earth. Bend your elbows and position your shin, right below the knee, on the upper arms.

3

Gaze slightly forward to encourage moving forward.

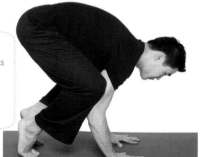

On an exhale, rock your weight forward. Begin to lift up on your toes, further planting your knees on the back of your upper arms above the elbows.

The goal is to place the fleshy part of the upper arm along the leg just below the knee. Things will be more difficult, and possibly uncomfortable or damaging to joints, if you place the elbow joint on knee joint. Take time to get this position down.

Begin the pose with your toes on blocks. This will give you a perch or launching pad and will allow for extra space to find your arm and leg positions.

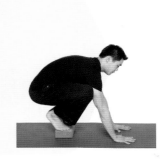

4

Keep your gaze steady. If you gaze down you'll encourage your body to drift down!

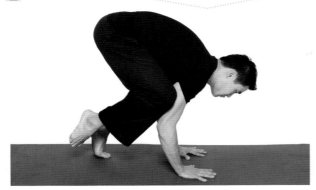

Lift one foot off the mat, using core strength.

5

Push into the earth with your hands.

On an exhale, rock forward, and bring your other foot off the mat. Think of squeezing through the pelvic floor and core. Gaze forward.

release   To release, simply rock back, bringing your toes to the mat.

Side Crow

Side Crow (*Bakasana*) takes Crow Pose and literally turns it to the side. Side Crow strengthens the arms and core, stretches the back, and builds confidence and balance.

SKILL LEVEL
●●●●●

1

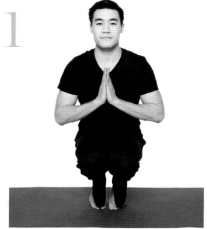

Begin in Tiptoe Squat, hands together in front of your heart.

2

This will be your base.

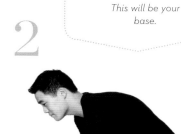

Bring your hands to the right and plant them on the mat, fingers spread wide.

3

Think of centering your heart toward the floor as much as possible.

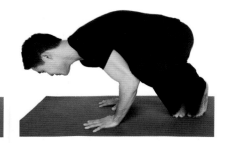

Lean forward and bend your elbows to make a shelf for your legs.

For a more stable base, you can use both upper arms as shelves instead of just one. Allow the outside of your thigh to rest on both arms. You will be creating an "H shape." Ideally, your thighs will stack on top of each other. Continue to gaze forward.

As you rock your weight forward to prepare for balance, gaze forward. If you look only down you may go down!

The inside bent leg rests on the outside bent elbow.

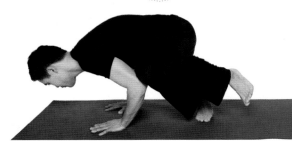

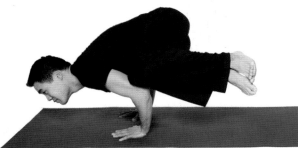

Come up on your tiptoes. Bring your right thigh to the top of your left tricep above the elbow. On an exhale begin to move forward, shifting weight from feet to hands.

Lift both of your feet, gazing forward. It's fine to start with just one foot lifted, as well! Press into your hands.

release   To release, gently bring the toes back to the mat on an exhale.

Wheel

Wheel Pose (*Urdhva Dhanurasana*) is sometimes also called Upward Bow. This pose is a large heart-opener, stretching the complete front of the body. Wheel is very energizing; don't try it just before bed! This pose can aid in fighting depression, stimulates the thyroid, and stretches the chest and lungs. Avoid if you have a serious back injury or migraine headache.

SKILL LEVEL
●●●●●

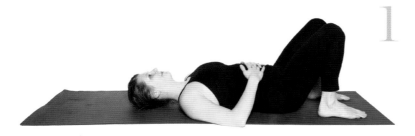

1 Begin by lying flat on the floor with knees bent and hands on your belly.

If you reach down with your hands, you want your fingertips to brush against your heels.

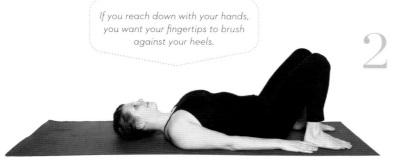

2 Draw your heels closer to your seat.

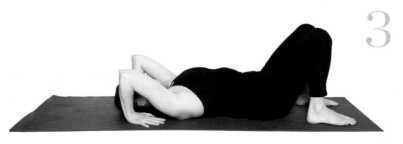

3 Bring your hands to rest by your ears, with fingers pointing toward the feet. Take a big breath in to prepare.

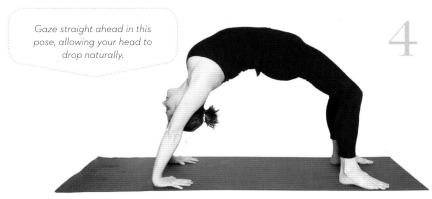

Gaze straight ahead in this pose, allowing your head to drop naturally.

4 On the exhale, push into the earth with your feet and hands. Raise your torso toward the sky.

variation

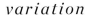

For an advanced variation, try pressing into the earth with both hands and one foot, then lifting the other foot. Point your toes to the ceiling.

Bridge Pose is a wonderful alternative for days you do not feel like coming up into full Wheel. Keep your hands by your hips and press your torso toward the sky.

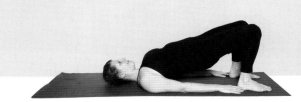

release To release, tuck your chin in toward your chest, then roll down on your back slowly. Be sure to always tuck the chin first to avoid dropping on your head and injuring your neck.

Headstand

Headstand (*Sirsasana*) is a powerful pose often referred to as the "King of Asanas." This posture calms the mind while strengthening the legs, arms, and core. It stimulates the pituitary and pineal glands and reverses blood flow in the body which can be therapeutic and rejuvenating. Avoid if you are menstruating, or have a neck injury or high blood pressure. This pose is best for those who have been practicing a while.

SKILL LEVEL
● ● ● ● ●

1

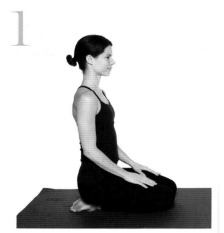

Begin in Hero's Pose, palms resting face-down on your thighs.

2

Front view of interlaced fingers.

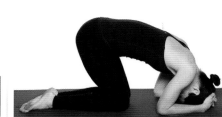

Come down onto bent elbows and interlace your fingers. Your elbows should be forearm's width apart.

3

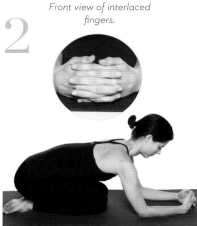

Bring the crown of your head to rest inside your hands, with hands cradling the upper back of your head.

keep it easy

When you are first learning this pose, it's great to practice near a wall. It should be just behind your back so if you need to, you can momentarily rest your heels against it, regain balance, and try alignment again.

Work your way up to staying in this pose for five minutes. You may wish to begin in this pose just for a few seconds, but work to increase endurance.

4

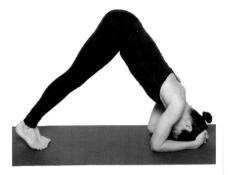

Curl your toes under, then straighten your legs.

5

Make sure your shoulders and hips are in a straight line.

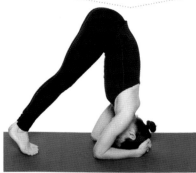

Walk your legs in closer toward your body.

6

Gaze straight ahead. Do not move the head from side to side. This could hurt the neck.

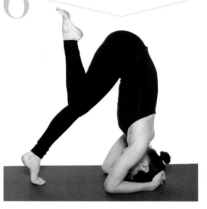

Using your core muscles, begin to bring one leg up off the floor ...

7

Begin to press into the earth with your hands and forearms, lifting your shoulders away from your ears.

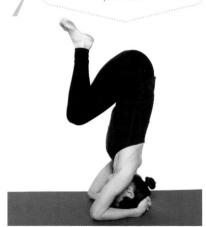

... then bend your other leg, bringing it up to meet the first.

8

It is very important not to fling yourself up! It's tempting, but can be dangerous.

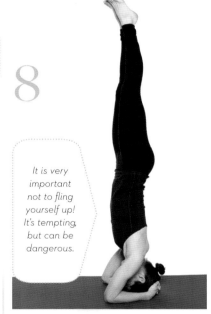

Continue to use your core, and extend your legs straight, aligned over your shoulders. Flex your feet.

release

Release from Headstand carefully. Use your core to curl your knees into your chest. Bring your toes to the earth, then relax into Child's Pose. When you are ready, slowly roll up to sit.

advanced poses   197

Smile, breathe and go slowly.

-Thich Nhat Hanh

MORE YOGA TECHNIQUES

The Eight Limbs of Yoga

When many of us think of yoga we think first of poses. But poses (or *asanas* in Sanskrit) make up only one branch out of the 8 limbs of yoga. Here we will explore all the limbs, or paths, as laid out by Patanjali in the *Yoga Sutras* thousands of years ago.

The eight limbs can be pictured as limbs of a tree. Together, these practices and philosophies are meant to help people live happy, healthy, peaceful lives. Like a tree, through the limbs we become strong yet flexible—connected to the earth yet also connected to the sky and heavens above.

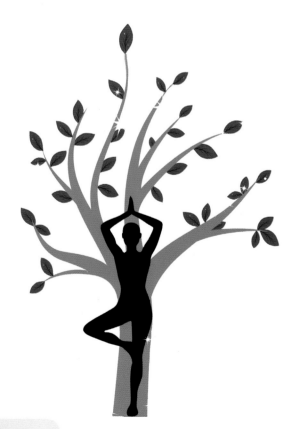

1. Yamas

The first limb, *yamas,* addresses how we interact ethically with the world around us. *Yamas* are all about personal conduct meant to guide us toward more harmonious living.

The five *yamas* are:

Ahimsa: nonviolence, avoiding harming

Satya: truthfulness

Asteya: non-stealing

Brahmacharya: self-restraint with regard to sexual activity; using creative energy wisely

Aparigraha: non-possessiveness, taking only what you need

There are many ways to think about and observe these *yamas.* You may choose to focus on *satya* for awhile, for example, working to be honest and truthful in all interactions. Many yogis approach vegetarianism from the idea of *ahimsa,* or nonviolence, toward the animals involved.

2. Niyama

Niyama, the second limb, has to do with how you relate to, and treat, yourself. *Niyamas* are all about cultivating internal harmony through certain behaviors.

The five *niyamas* are:

Saucha: cleanliness

Santosha: contentment; being satisfied with what you have

Tapas: good discipline, such as maintaining a yoga practice

Svadhyaya: study of the self through meditation and other means

Ishvara Pranidhana: devotion; sense of surrender toward the divine

3. Asana

Asanas, the postures practiced in yoga, comprise the third limb. In the yogic point of view, the body is a temple of spirit. Through *asanas* we take good care of our health in body, mind, and spirit at the same time. We develop flexibility, strength, balance, mindfulness, and the intimacy of knowing ourselves from the inside out. In traditional yoga, *asanas* also helped to prepare the body for sitting meditation.

4. Pranayama

This branch consists of breath work. Through getting to know our breath and how to use it to energize and de-stress, we gain mastery over our emotions and bodies in a way that is not forceful but, instead, works with the body. In short, *pranayama* leads to a steady mind. We also gain an energetic awareness of ourselves.

5. Pratyahara

Pratyahara, the fifth limb, means withdrawal of the senses. In this branch we begin to draw attention and energy inside instead of being swept away by external stimuli. We become very aware of our senses—not denying them but focusing more within.

One easy way to begin exploring *pratyahara* is in Corpse Pose (*Savasana*). When you lie on your back with eyes closed, usually at the end of yoga practice, let the breath be natural and focus on how you feel. You are still in touch with the outside world: you know you are lying on a mat, you may notice how the air feels, but your attention is more inside yourself than outside.

6. Dharana

The practice of *pratyahara* prepares us for *dharana,* or concentration. Now that we're looking within, we begin to deal with the distractions of the mind itself. In this branch we focus on one thing at a time. This practice builds inner muscles which lead to meditation.

Dharana is the opposite of multi-tasking. Think of it as focusing on one thing thoroughly, without hopping to something else.

7. Dhyana

In the yoga tradition, *dhyana* (meditation) is the uninterrupted flow of soft but steady concentration. Here we begin to experience stillness beyond the fluctuations of the mind.

8. Samadhi

Samadhi is described as a state of bliss. At this stage, the yogi merges with his or her point of focus and transcends the individual self. The yogi may feel a strong connection to the divine and to all living beings. This feeling can help us understand how we are all connected and that the actions and thoughts of the individual affect the whole. This is considered to be a sense of peace brought about by action and which will inspire more action.

Mindful Eating

Mindful eating is the practice of becoming aware of the experience of eating and really noticing how food makes you feel. Instead of multi-tasking while eating (reading, talking, surfing the internet, or watching TV), with this practice you are guided to just focus on eating. Chances are you eat several times a day, so with the practice of mindful eating you have many chances to practice presence, awareness, compassion, and attention!

One of my first experiences with mindful eating was on a meditation retreat with Zen teacher Thich Nhat Hahn. For meals we ate in silence, paying attention to the texture, taste, and affect of the foods we were enjoying. At first it felt a little awkward to sit with others and eat without talking. Then, it became very peaceful and nourishing. I felt I was enjoying and digesting everything better.

The practice of mindful eating can help us tune in to our bodies. Through these approaches we can develop healthy relationships to food. We are also giving thanks for nourishment.

Techniques to Try

Silent Eating—Turn off the TV, the internet, and silence your cell phone. Give food your full attention. This can be uncomfortable at first! Notice the itch you may feel to grab for a magazine or friend. See if you can pay attention to the tastes, sensations, and purposes of each bite. Notice when your satiety cues chime in, telling you you've had enough to eat. Notice how you physically and emotionally feel about the food you are eating, but without judgment. Instead, approach the whole practice with gratitude and curiosity.

Slow Down Eating—Many of us habitually race through meals to get to the next task at hand. See if you can practice a slow meal, taking the time to really enjoy the food offered. Perhaps you will chew more than normal, or pause between bites to savor the tastes and prepare yourself for more. If we eat slower, our bodies have a better chance to tell us when we are full.

You may want to start with one mindful meal a week, working your way up in frequency. Connecting with food in a loving way is a wonderful gift to our bodies and psyches, especially in this time of rushed and disordered eating. Through this practice we can not only give thanks for nourishment but can begin to hear more of what our bodies need!

Mudras

I like to think of mudras as yoga for your hands. Mudras are used in poses and in seated meditation. But these gestures can also be used, "off the mat" in daily life when you need to connect with the meaning they impart. You can, for example, quickly do a chin mudra when walking down the street if you need to remind yourself you are taken care of by the world, and are part of it yourself. I often consider whether my palms are open, in a gesture of receptivity, or faced downward, in a grounded gesture, when simply sitting. Awareness of hands in this way can quickly connect you to heart.

Mudra translates to "seal" in Sanskrit. Most mudras involve the hands and fingers and are said to seal in energy to create a spiritual, meaningful gesture. Some yoga poses can be considered full body mudras that seal in energy in new ways. Here we explore some popular and easy-to-use hand mudras.

Abhaya Mudra

Abhaya translates to "fearlessness" in Sanskrit. To practice, place your right hand up with the palm facing forward. Place your left hand on your thigh either with palm down or up. The right palm, facing open and forward, represents a gesture of openness. There is no weapon in the hand; no object of protection. This open hand represents fearlessness and peace. I also think of this open palm as a gesture of being open, in a fearless way, to what is to come.

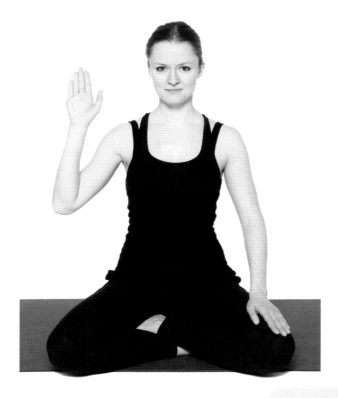

Anjali Mudra

Anjali translates as "to offer" in Sanskrit, and this *mudra* is a gesture of honoring. It is also known as "prayer hands." Here we bring the right and left palms to touch with all fingers pointing upward, often with hands in front of the heart. Some yogis I know like to keep a small space in the palms to hold an intention, wish, or prayer. With hands in front of the heart, see if you can feel your heart beat against your thumbs.

In some settings this mudra is used as a gesture of saying hello or goodbye, with respect. Often *anjali mudra* is practiced with a small bow of the head. By bringing the right and left hands together we are also connecting the right and left sides of the brain to achieve union, or "yoking."

Chin Mudra

This is a very popular *mudra* often seen in Western yoga. To practice, connect your forefinger with your thumb. I like to have my thumb resting over the forefinger slightly. Keep the rest of the fingers extended open.

It is said the thumb represents the universe and the finger represents you, the individual. By taking this gesture you are reminding yourself that you, the individual, are part of the universe and the universe is taking care of you. This is a seal of union, a gesture of connection.

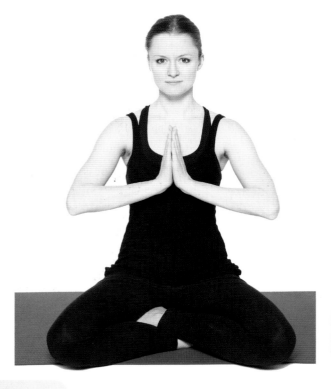

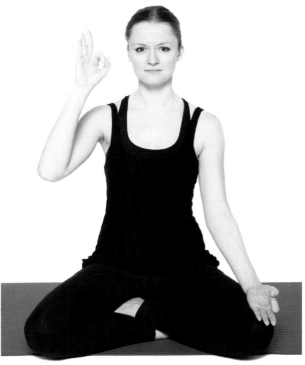

Dhyana Mudra

Dhyana translates to "meditation." It is a gesture of concentration often used in seated meditation practices. Sit with your hands just below your belly button. Usually the non-dominant hand rests on top of the dominant hand. Allow your fingers to rest on each other like a bowl. Bring your thumbs to gently touch. As you sit and meditate, these fingers can be a sort of thermometer of your attention. If your thumbs start to slack, you know you are losing your attentiveness. If your thumbs are pressing too hard into each other, you know you need to release and relax a bit. Sit and observe breath with this hand posture. Feel the freedom and space in the small bowl your hands are creating.

Hakini Mudra

Hakini mudra is a gesture of concentration. To practice, hold your hands in front of you with palms facing each other. Bring all of your fingertips to touch, so your hands form the shape of a tent. Allow the rest of your body to relax while maintaining an upright spine. Breathe! This *mudra* is said to naturally improve mental focus and the coordination between the left and right hemispheres. You may naturally see some people performing this *mudra* while giving speeches.

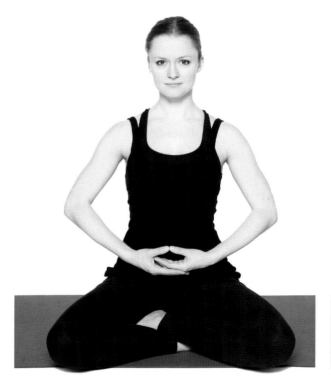

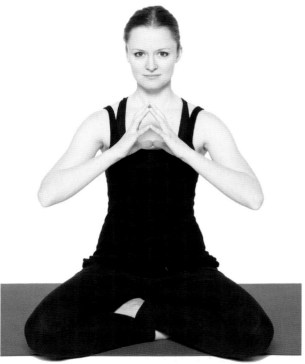

more yoga techniques

205

Mantras

Working with *mantras,* or repeated sounds or phrases, is another beneficial practice. *Mantra* is sometimes described as "mind protection" because the words are meant to redirect the mind (and spirit!) toward the positive and away from worry or negative thought. *Mantras* can work as a bridge to help us cross from worry to peace.

A *mantra* may appear as a single sound—a "seed *mantra*" such as *OM*—or it may be a phrase that is repeated. A *mantra* can be in any language, though many in the yoga tradition are in Sanskrit. Sanskrit is said to have a healing, melodic, and poetic energy that translates the meaning of the words in sound vibration. For example, *OM,* which roughly translates to "sound of the universe" or a unifying sound, requires three parts of the mouth's palate to sing. Therefore, it physically creates a unifying sensation in the mouth and body. The content mirrors the form. Having an English *mantra* is helpful as well. For example, "May I be happy," is a great English *mantra* to repeat. The main point is that the *mantra* sounds, and feels, uplifting to you.

Mantras appear in many traditions. In yoga practice, often *mantras* are sung or chanted. There are many wonderful recordings of *mantras* online and in digital format if you want to hear them sung but do not have a teacher or class near you. Using sound in your practice means bringing vibration into the body, and that itself is quite healing. Couple that with the positive and powerful meanings of *mantras* and you'll see why they are said to be keys to transformation.

Kirtan

If you enjoy the use of sound in your yoga practice, you may want to explore *kirtan. Kirtan* consists of devotional singing and is, therefore, considered a practice of *bhakti,* or devotion. I often play *kirtan* music (which can be found online or in CDs) whenever I need to feel more positive, upbeat, or connected. If you go to a *kirtan* event at your local yoga center you'll find it is usually presented in call-and-response style. Here, you and your voice are part of the song. Of course, if you are not comfortable singing you can simply take in the good vibrations!

Mantra Japa

Many who love *mantra* take on a *mantra japa* practice. This consists of using a *mala,* or a set of beads. In *japa* practice, a practitioner will say or chant a *mantra* over and over in a cycle, using the beads to help count. A *mala* has 108 beads and a guru bead, which is the head bead of the strand. Once a practitioner reaches the main bead, he or she may repeat or rest. *Mantra japa* is a complete practice in and of itself and helps many find a single point of focus in the mind. It is said that someone practicing *japa* finds unity with the idea of the *mantra.*

Some *Mantras* to Try

These mantras are taken from yoga traditions, Buddhist traditions, and even poetry. All can be used in your practice or daily life.

OM—A *bija* (seed) *mantra, OM* may be the most common *mantra* you'll encounter in yoga. Usually chanted three times, it is a very whole and complete sound meant to make us feel one with the universe around us. It is a sound (and feeling) of union. Note that *OM* is actually made of 4 parts and is sometimes spelled *AUM*. The 4 parts are: Ah, Ooh, MM, and the silence afterward.

SO HUM—I am that, That I am

Shanti, shanti, shanti—Peace, Peace, Peace

May I be happy, may I be free—This form of Loving Kindness *mantra* toward the self (from the Buddhist tradition) can also substitute "you" or "all" for "I."

In gladness and in safety, May all beings be at ease.—A form of Loving Kindness *mantra* toward all (from the Buddhist tradition).

Lokah samasta sukhino bhavantu—May all beings be happy and free, and may the thoughts, words, and actions of my own life contribute in some way to this happiness and freedom.

Maitri-adishu balani—Through compassion and love, strength comes. (From the *Yoga Sutras,* written down by Patanjali)

I am larger and better than I thought. I did not know I held so much goodness.—These words from American poet Walt Whitman can be used as a *mantra.*

Chakras

Chakras are energy centers in the body. The word *chakra* is derivative of the Sanskrit word for "wheel" or "turning," and indeed *chakras* are thought of as wheels of energy. The *chakra* are related to the energy we're radiating, the energy we are able to receive, and the way in which we process or digest energy around us.

While there are many *chakras*, in the Western world it is generally thought that there are 7 main *chakras* which run from the base of the spine upward. Some believe the lower six *chakra* points correspond to major centers of nerves in the body (nerve plexus). In this way, the physical is reflecting the energetic!

Each *chakra* is associated with a different color; seed syllable (sometimes used in mantra practice); and emotional, spiritual, and physical state.

Experiences, thoughts, and feelings can be reflected in the *chakras*. It is thought a blocked or compromised *chakra* will manifest in illness, injury, or disease. For example, if you are dealing with chronic laryngitis—losing your voice—you may want to look at the emotional and energetic issues of the throat *chakra*. The physical manifestation of an issue may be the reflection of other imbalances in this area. By connecting with the seed syllable or color you can help balance and purify the associated *chakra*. It is worthwhile to strive for balance. Through *chakra* study, we can work toward this.

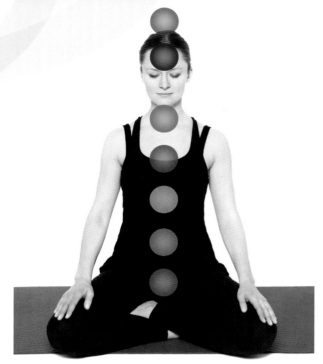

Muladhara: The Root Chakra

Concerns: foundation and sense of groundedness; feeling safe; having basic needs covered and cared for; survival; fight or flight response; stability

Color: Red

Location: Base of spine

Seed syllable: *Lam*

Svadhisthana: The Sacral Chakra

Concerns: connection to others; sexuality; creativity; reproductive system; addictions; basic emotional needs; pleasure

Color: Orange

Location: Below the navel

Seed syllable: *Vam*

Manipura: The Solar Plexus Chakra

Concerns: confidence; digestive system; personal power; decision making; self-esteem

Color: Yellow

Location: Abdomen

Seed syllable: *Ram*

Anahata: The Heart Chakra

Concerns: love; compassion; ability to embrace life

Color: Green

Location: Heart center (center of chest)

Seed syllable: *Yam*

Vishuddha: The Throat Chakra

Concerns: communication and expression; thyroid function; speaking up for yourself

Color: Blue

Location: Throat

Seed syllable: *Ham*

Ajna: The Brow Chakra

Concerns: intuition; trusting your inner guidance; vision

Color: Purple

Location: Third eye (space between and just above eyebrows)

Seed syllable: *OM*

Sahasrara: The Crown Chakra

Concerns: connection with the divine; sense of sacredness

Color: Indigo

Location: Just above the head; sometimes the crown of the head

Seed syllable: *OM*

To connect with a certain *chakra*, sit in Easy Seat and chant or sing the seed syllable while focusing your attention on that particular energy center. You can also wear, decorate, or otherwise surround yourself with the color associated with the *chakra*. In a seated meditation you may choose to visualize the color associated with the *chakra* radiating in and out of the related body area. You may also simply contemplate the area of your life and the concerns the *chakra* governs. This should be done with curiosity and compassion, not judgment! The *asana* practice works to balance our *chakras* naturally.

The idea is that as we develop we move from basic security at the root of our beings, up through connection with others and sexuality, to confidence and personal power, then develop toward love and compassion, voice and expression, and intuition and a connection to the divine. At different stages of our lives we may be focused on one part more than another. Various situations, also, may touch upon different energy centers. By adulthood, it is hoped that the *chakra* are all activated and we can work daily to stay balanced through reflection, yoga pose practice, and taking good care of ourselves.

Seated Meditation

It's possible to use your pose practice as a moving meditation—a way to settle into silence—but yoga poses were also meant to help your body prepare for seated meditation. Sitting for long periods of time can be physically trying as well as mentally and emotionally tricky. Ancient yogis often used Downward Facing Dog and Cobra Pose to get ready for seated meditation.

Sitting in tune with your breath and mind can help you get to know yourself in profound ways. It can rewire the brain's reaction to stress and provide insight into the changing nature of life. Everything arises, then passes away—from thoughts and breath to jobs and relationships. Learning to sit and stay calm with change is huge! Meditation is also a way to release toxic stress from the body and mind.

Benefits

This meditation trains the mind to be both sensitive and steady (much like the state of the body in yoga!), allowing for less reactivity, a more even response to stress, and an awareness of the present moment.

Practice staying in the present moment. We often dwell in the past or worry about the future. Training the mind (and it takes training!) to stay more present is an instant release of those two kinds of suffering.

Posture

Finding comfort in a long-term seat can be harder than it sounds! The idea is to have a seated position that supports your practice. You want to be upright and alert, but with ease.

Try sitting on a folded blanket, pillow, or cushion. You may want to invest in a zafu, which is a sitting meditation cushion. The idea is to have your hips above your knees to aid in the proper tilt of the pelvis so your spine can be upright. Allow your shoulders to roll away from your ears. Sit so your chin is parallel with the earth. You can use Easy Seat as a model.

Hands

Take a moment to consider hand placement. Palms down on the thighs is a gesture of calm abiding. This hand position will send the message to your mind and body to observe in a grounded way.

If you are looking to evoke a gesture of receptivity, sit with palms open to the sky, with the backs of the hands resting on the legs.

You may also want to sit with one of the *mudras*, like *dhyana mudra*. This shape is common in Zen meditation. It takes a gentle alertness to maintain this hand position. If you find your thumbs are slumping, this is a message to your mind to wake up! If you find your thumbs are pressing together too hard, this is a reminder to relax a bit.

Basic Breath Awareness Meditation

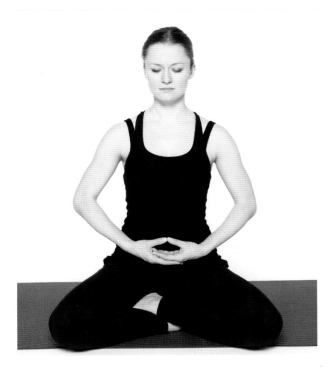

Here is a simple breath meditation you can explore now. Aim to practice your seated meditation on a regular basis. The benefits of meditation reveal themselves most over time and with practice. Start with just 10 minutes a day and see if you can work your way up to 30. Many people like to sit first thing in the morning, to check in with themselves and establish equanimity of mind before the day begins. An afternoon sit or end-of-day session provide different benefits, perhaps helping to clear your mind and provide focus in your tasks. You can also sit after your yoga practice when your body and mind are feeling open and good.

Step 1: Scan the body. Be aware of any held tension and see, with an exhale, if you can release it.

Step 2: Find the sensation of breath in your body as you breathe naturally. You may feel it in your chest or throat, or perhaps you can feel the breath moving in and out of your nose, brushing over the bit of skin above the upper lip and below the nostrils. Simply feel the breath.

Step 3: Track the breath. There are several ways to do this. You may wish to feel the sensation of breathing. Or you may silently label "inhale" and "exhale" with each breath. You may count your breath from 1 to 5, then start over again. The important thing is to work with your mind to focus on breathing. Simple—but a challenge!

Step 4: Inevitably, you'll find yourself thinking about anything *but* breath. The mind loves to drift, float, and think up problems to solve. This is just what the mind does. The mind that jumps from thought to thought instead of staying with the breath is called Monkey Mind in some Buddhist circles. When you notice you've drifted, simply redirect your attention back to your breath!

It is not a moment of failure when you see your mind has drifted into daydreams, worry, etc. Actually, that moment you notice your mind is doing something other than following breath is a moment you "woke up!" It's a helpful moment. Just label it "thinking" and come back to "breathing." You may find yourself doing this for your whole meditation session. That's okay. With time—like working out a muscle—your focus will increase so you are spending less time redirecting and more time being.

Notice how sitting with regularity changes your mood and mind in day-to-day life.

We are not going to change the whole world, but we can change ourselves and feel free as birds. We can be serene even in the midst of calamities and, by our serenity, make others more tranquil. Serenity is contagious.

—Swami Satchidananda

SEQUENCES

In this section, we'll take the poses we've learned and put them together in short "flows" or routines. You will move with breath, flowing from one pose to the next without stopping in between. See if you can pay attention to the transitions between poses as much as the poses themselves, infusing all of your movement (and stillness!) with the quality of paying attention.

A note on breath: You'll notice as you go, unless otherwise noted, poses are moved into on inhales, and exited on exhales. 3 breaths means full breath cycles (complete inhale/full exhale, inhale/exhale, inhale/exhale). The number of breaths in each pose is a suggestion; if you would like to stay longer that's fine, if you prefer to leave the pose sooner just be aware of your exit. Think of each breath cycle as complete and composed of three parts: the inhale, the slight hold at the top of the breath, and the complete exhale. Allow your shapes and your movements between them to be filled with breath awareness.

A note on poses: When a pose is suggested, feel free to try the beginner variation or a more advanced variation. Yogi's choice!

The sequences are meant to be prescriptive. If you have back pain, you can try the back pain sequence for relief. If you are having trouble sleeping, try the bedtime flow. But notice how you, in particular, feel as you try these routines. You may think of even more situations in which you'd like to try these sequences!

Sun Salutation A

Sun Salutation A (*Surya Namaskar A*) is an ancient sequence that is a salute to, or greeting toward, the sun. It will warm up your body like the sun warms the earth. Most people find this sequence to be mentally, spiritually, and physically enlivening. It is a complete cycle, meaning once you get to the end you can start over and complete several times. I recommend at least three Sun Salutations to really connect breath with movement and mind with breath.

Note: Unless stated, you will inhale with one pose and exhale with the next. If this feels too speedy as you learn, you can take one breath cycle per pose.

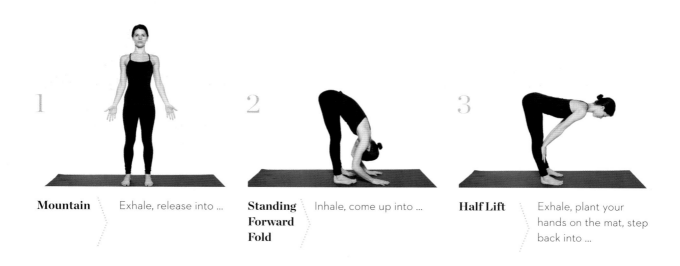

Mountain — Exhale, release into ...

Standing Forward Fold — Inhale, come up into ...

Half Lift — Exhale, plant your hands on the mat, step back into ...

4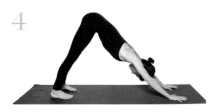

Downward Facing Dog
3-5 breaths

Exhale into ...

5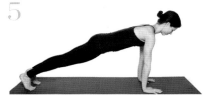

Plank
1 breath

Exhale, lower into ...

6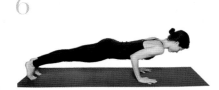

Chuturanga

Exhale down to the mat, inhale up into ...

Advanced yogis can replace Cobra with Upward Facing Dog.

7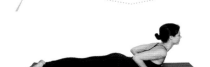

Cobra

Exhale, push back onto your knees, bringing your seat to your heels into ...

8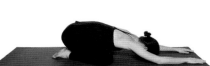

Child's Pose

Inhale, extend into...

9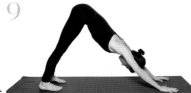

Downward Facing Dog
3-5 breaths

Step your feet forward between your hands, release into ...

10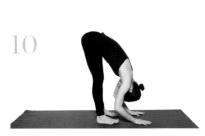

Standing Forward Fold

Inhale and roll up into ...

11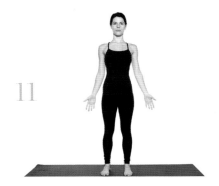

Mountain
3-5 breaths

Sun Salutation B

Sun Salutation B is another classic yoga sequence you may encounter in a class (but it's also great to practice on your own, outside of a class). Do your best to move through the shapes, one breath per movement. We will inhale with one shape and exhale with the next. If this feels too speedy, you can take one full cycle of breath per pose.

Sun Salutation B is a bit longer than Sun Salutation A, but is also wonderful to do in sets of at least 3. This will warm up your body and mind. You may find the rhythm to be soothing and enlivening at the same time.

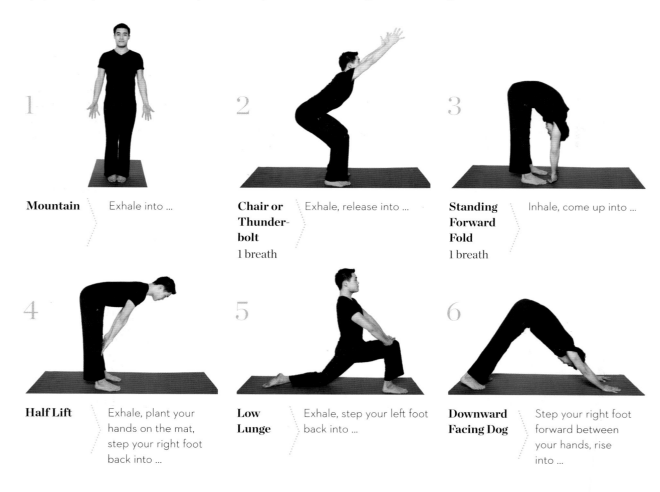

1

Mountain   Exhale into ...

2

Chair or Thunder-bolt
1 breath   Exhale, release into ...

3

Standing Forward Fold
1 breath   Inhale, come up into ...

4

Half Lift   Exhale, plant your hands on the mat, step your right foot back into ...

5

Low Lunge   Exhale, step your left foot back into ...

6

Downward Facing Dog   Step your right foot forward between your hands, rise into ...

7

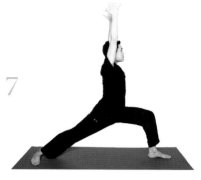

Warrior 1   Exhale, bring your hands down to the mat, step back into ...

8

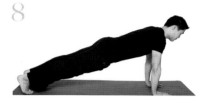

Plank
1 breath   Exhale into ...

9

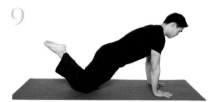

Chuturanga   Inhale into ...

10

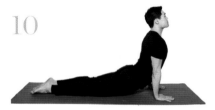

Cobra or Upward Facing Dog   Exhale, bring your seat to your heels, extend into ...

11

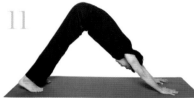

Downward Facing Dog   Exhale, step your left foot forward in a low lunge ...

12

Repeat Warrior 1 on left side, Plank, Chuturanga, Cobra or Upward Facing Dog, and Downward Facing Dog. By the end of this cycle you should have done this "flow" on both sides of the body.

Repeat   Bring your feet forward to your hands, release into ...

13

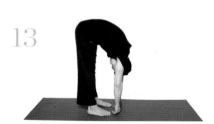

Standing Forward Fold   Exhale, sit back into ...

14

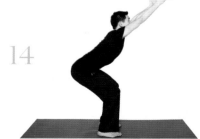

Chair   Inhale, press up into ...

15

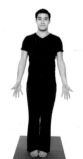

Mountain
3-5 breaths

Fatigue

This sequence is designed to allow you to first acknowledge how you are feeling, then begin to bring fresh breath and increased blood flow into the body to gently awaken it. Taking the time to do this sequence when you are tired will lead to invigoration that is more natural and longer lasting than a shot of espresso. Be sure to start near a wall, for the Legs Up the Wall Pose toward the end of the sequence.

1

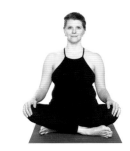

Easy Seat
3-5 breaths

Come onto your hands and knees, walk your hands toward your feet, come into ...

2

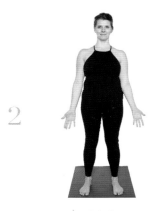

Mountain
3-5 breaths

Exhale into ...

3

Inhale to center, exhale into the right side.

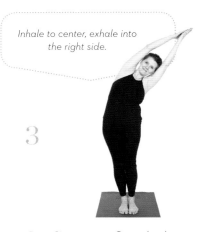

Standing Side Stretch
3 breaths on each side

Come back to center, release into ...

4

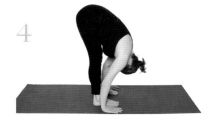

Standing Forward Fold
3 breaths

Plant your hands on the mat, step back into ...

5

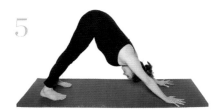

Downward Dog
5 breaths

Exhale, step your right foot forward into ...

6

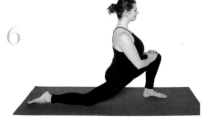

Low Lunge
5-8 breaths on each side

Plant your hands on the mat, come into ...

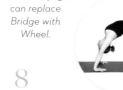

Advanced yogis can replace Bridge with Wheel.

7

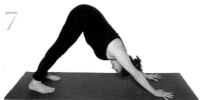

Downward Facing Dog
5 breaths

Come onto all fours, bring your seat onto the mat, lie down and move into ...

8

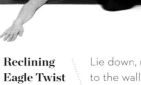

Bridge
5 breaths, rest, 5 breaths again

Lie down on the mat, arms and legs extended, move into ...

9

Reclining Eagle Twist
5-8 breaths on each side

Lie down, move over to the wall and move into ...

10

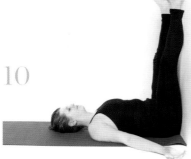

Legs Up the Wall
1-3 minutes

Move away from the wall, extend into ...

11

Corpse
At least 5 minutes

Back Pain

Many people hold stress in different parts of the back, and long periods of sitting at a computer or office desk can add to common back woes. This sequence is designed to stretch and relieve pain, but also works to strengthen the core of the body. A strong core equals a stronger and healthier back in the long run.

For a variation, you can alternate Cat and Cow in one breath cycle—inhale into Cat, exhale into Cow.

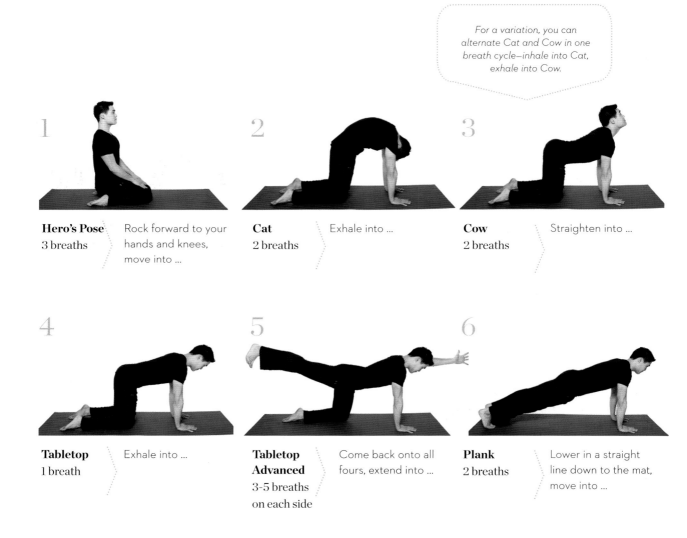

1

Hero's Pose
3 breaths

Rock forward to your hands and knees, move into ...

2

Cat
2 breaths

Exhale into ...

3

Cow
2 breaths

Straighten into ...

4

Tabletop
1 breath

Exhale into ...

5

Tabletop Advanced
3-5 breaths on each side

Come back onto all fours, extend into ...

6

Plank
2 breaths

Lower in a straight line down to the mat, move into ...

7

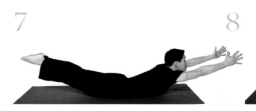

Superhero
3-5 breaths

> Come down onto
> your belly, flip onto
> your back, and come
> up into ...

8

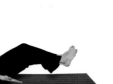

Boat
3-5 breaths

> Extend down to lie
> on the mat, move
> into ...

9

**Reclining
Eagle Twist**
5-8 breaths on
each side

> Come back to center,
> extend arms and legs
> into ...

10

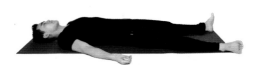

Corpse
At least 5
minutes

Anxiety

Yoga is a powerful tool to deal with anxiety. The purpose of this sequence is to soothe the mind and the nervous system, imparting a true sense of calm. By following this flow, you will cool down your system, ground yourself, and reconnect to the here and now through breath awareness.

1

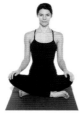

Easy Seat
3 breaths

Rock forward on your knees, place your hands on the floor, uncross your legs, and move into ...

2

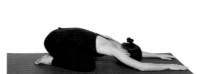

Child's Pose
5 breaths

Come up onto your hands and knees, and move into ...

3

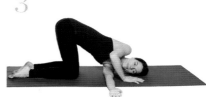

Thread the Needle
3 breaths on each side

Come up onto your hands and knees, step one foot in and slowly come to standing. Move into ...

4

Mountain
3 breaths

Slowly roll forward into ...

5

Standing Forward Fold
3 breaths

Come up into ...

6

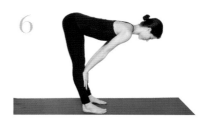

Half Lift
1 breath

Exhale, place your hands on the floor, step back into ...

Advanced yogis can replace Cobra with Upward Facing Dog.

7

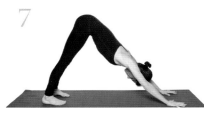

Downward Facing Dog
5 breaths

Exhale, roll your weight forward into ...

8

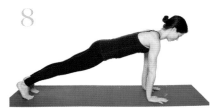

Plank
2 breaths

Exhale and carefully lower down in one straight line into ...

9

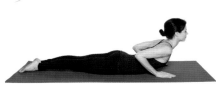

Cobra
3 breaths

Exhale, push into the mat with your hands. Come back into a momentary Child's Pose, then up into ...

10

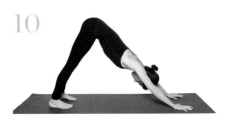

Downward Facing Dog
5 breaths

Walk your hands back toward your feet and find your ...

11

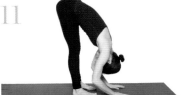

Standing Forward Fold
2 breaths

Roll up into ...

12

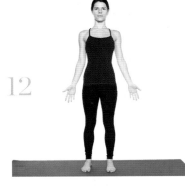

Mountain
3 breaths

Cross your feet at the ankles, and lower down to the floor carefully, coming to sit in ...

13

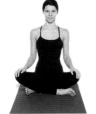

Easy Seat
2 breaths

Uncross and extend your legs while you roll back into ...

14

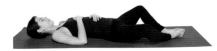

Goddess
5-8 breaths

Extend your arms and legs into ...

15

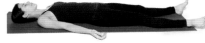

Corpse
At least
5 minutes

Tighten and Tone

If you're looking for a sequence that's more of a "workout" this is
your flow! Since we use our own body weight to develop strength
in yoga, you'll never develop bulk—just tone. And as you are increas-
ingly able to "hold your own weight" you will feel mentally stronger and
more confident, too.

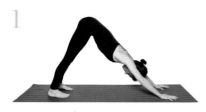

**Downward
Facing Dog**

5 breaths

Extend into ...

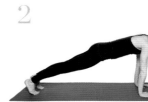

Plank

3-5 breaths

Repeat Downward Facing Dog
and Plank 3 times, one breath/one
movement (inhale into Plank, exhale into Downward Facing Dog).
Step your right foot forward,
moving into ...

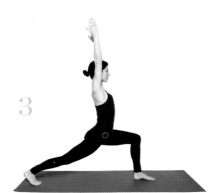

High Lunge

3-5 breaths

Lower your left heel
to the mat and open
your hips to the side,
transitioning into ...

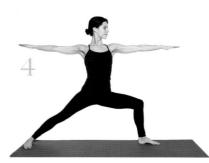

Warrior 2

3-5 breaths

Step forward into Mountain, stay for
1 breath, then step your right foot
back and repeat High Lunge and
Warrior 2 on the other side. Come
forward into Mountain, move into ...

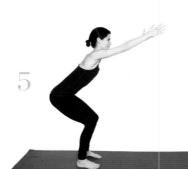

5

Chair

3-5 breaths

Bring your feet together, move into ...

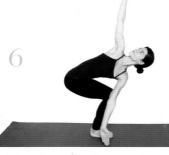

6

Thunder-bolt Twist

3-5 breaths

on each side

Come back into Chair, release into ...

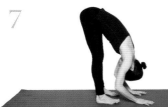

7

Standing Forward Fold

3-5 breaths

Plant your hands on the mat, step back into ...

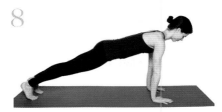

8

Plank

3 breaths

Lower your body to the mat, flip onto your back and move into ...

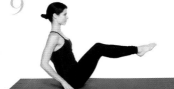

9

Boat

3-5 breaths

Feel free to repeat Boat up to 3 times. Release into ...

10

Corpse

At least 5 minutes

sequences 225

Strengthen Your Core

This sequence is not about simply having strong abs and spine, but also a strong and stable sense of self. All yoga poses reach and radiate from the core of our bodies. Most of us hope our actions, thoughts, and words radiate from the core of our beings as well. For these reasons it's important to get in touch with our centers.

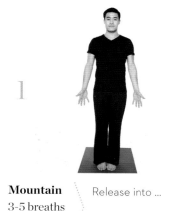

1

Mountain
3-5 breaths

Release into ...

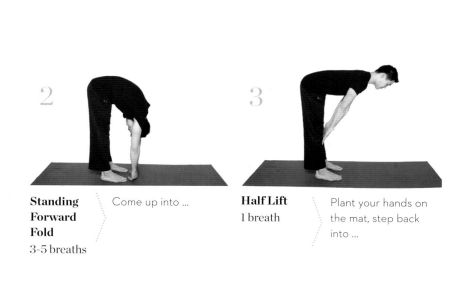

2

**Standing
Forward
Fold**
3-5 breaths

Come up into ...

3

Half Lift
1 breath

Plant your hands on
the mat, step back
into ...

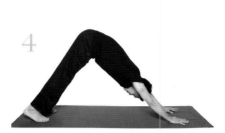

4

Downward Facing Dog
5 breaths

Bring the right leg up into ...

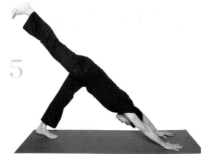

5

Three-Legged Dog
3 breaths on each side

Come into Downward Facing Dog, extend into ...

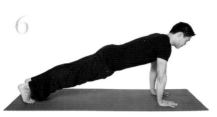

6

Plank
3-5 breaths

Bring your right hand to the center of your body, transition into ...

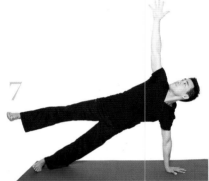

7

Side Plank
5-8 breaths on each side

Come back into Plank, lower onto your forearms and into ...

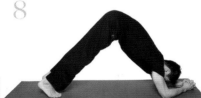

8

Dolphin
5 breaths

Plant your hands on the mat, lower your belly to the mat and move into ...

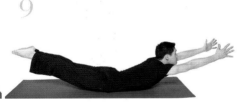

9

Superhero
3-5 breaths

Lower onto your belly, flip onto your back, come into ...

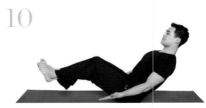

10

Boat
5-8 breaths

Lower onto the mat, extend into ...

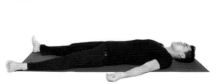

11

Corpse
At least 5 minutes

Hear Yourself Think

Whether your mind is over-active or a little sluggish, this sequence is designed to help you drop the stress and fatigue that can clutter thoughts. If you find yourself tempted to say, "I can't hear myself think!" try dropping into all or part of this sequence. Be sure you start near a wall, for the Legs Up the Wall Pose toward the end of the sequence.

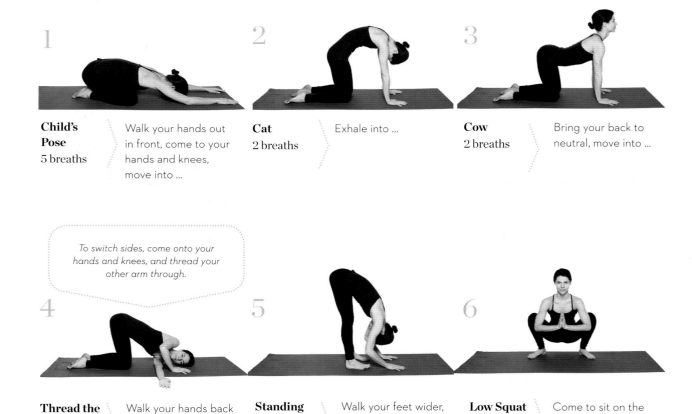

1

Child's Pose
5 breaths

Walk your hands out in front, come to your hands and knees, move into ...

2

Cat
2 breaths

Exhale into ...

3

Cow
2 breaths

Bring your back to neutral, move into ...

To switch sides, come onto your hands and knees, and thread your other arm through.

4

Thread the Needle
5-8 breaths on each side

Walk your hands back to your feet, relax into ...

5

Standing Forward Fold
3-5 breaths

Walk your feet wider, lower your seat into ...

6

Low Squat
5-8 breaths

Come to sit on the mat, extend your legs into ...

To change sides, push back into Downward Facing Dog, then step your left foot forward.

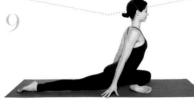

7

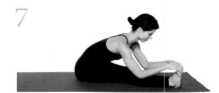

Seated Two Leg Forward Fold
5-8 breaths

Bend your knees into Easy Seat, walk your hands in front of you, extend into ...

8

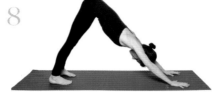

Downward Facing Dog
5 breaths

Step your right foot forward, move into ...

9

Pigeon
8 breaths on each side

Bring your leg back. Come onto your hands and knees, sit down on the mat, extend your right leg into ...

10

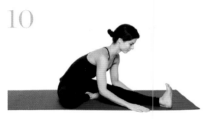

Seated One Leg Forward Fold
5-8 breaths on each side

Bring the soles of your feet to touch, lie back into ...

11

Goddess
8-10 breaths

Slowly bring your knees together, move to the wall and into ...

12

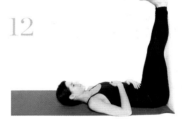

Legs Up the Wall
1-3 minutes

Move away from the wall, extend into ...

13

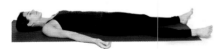

Corpse
At least 5 minutes

Morning

Wake up your body, mind, and spirit with a morning routine! This sequence will set a peaceful, caring tone of awareness for the day. As you move through the poses below, allow yourself to notice how you are feeling and perhaps take the time to set an intention for the day, or practice some gratitude for the fresh start of a new morning.

1

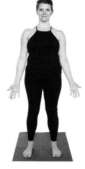

Mountain
3-5 breaths

Inhale your arms over your head, exhale into ...

2

Standing Side Stretch
3-5 breaths on each side

Come back into Mountain, step your left leg back, move into ...

3

Triangle
3 breaths

Exhale, bring your torso upright, move into ...

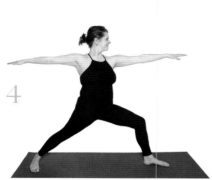

Warrior 2
3 breaths

Exhale into ...

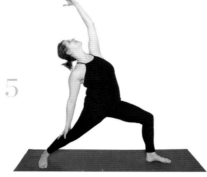

Peaceful Warrior
3 breaths

Come back into Warrior 2, switch sides, and repeat Triangle, Warrior 2, and Peaceful Warrior on the left side. Release, step into Mountain, move into ...

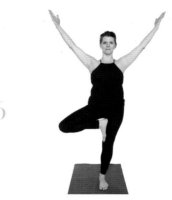

Tree
5 breaths on each side

Come back into Mountain, move into ...

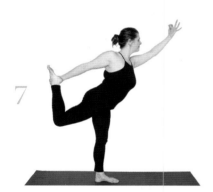

Dancer
5 breaths on each side

Come to standing, cross your feet, sit into Easy Seat, move into ...

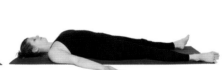

Reclining Hero
8-10 breaths

Extend your feet, lie down into ...

Corpse
At least 5 minutes

Bedtime

This bedtime flow is designed to help you soothe the mind and body in preparation for a deep and restorative sleep. Allow yourself the time to go through this sequence to release any remaining tension, mental or physical, from your day.

1

Child's Pose
3-5 breaths

Walk your hands out in front, extend to lie on your belly and move into ...

2

Cobra
3-5 breaths

Tuck your toes under, push your seat to your heels, extend back into ...

3

Downward Facing Dog
5-8 breaths

Step the right foot forward, move into ...

To change between sides for Pigeon, push back into Downward Facing Dog, then step the left foot forward, and move into the pose.

4

Pigeon
8-10 breaths on each side

Release your left leg, come onto hands and knees, exhale into ...

5

Cat
2 breaths

Exhale into ...

6

Cow
2 breaths

Come back to sit on the mat, bring your legs in front of you, move into ...

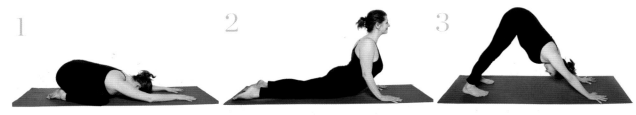

7

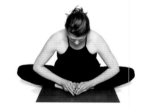

Butterfly
5 breaths

> Roll back to lie down on the mat, move into ...

8

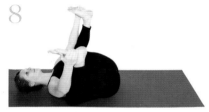

Happy Baby
5 breaths

> Lie back on the mat, release the legs and arms, move into ...

9

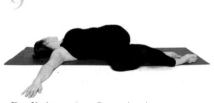

Reclining Eagle Twist
5-8 breaths on each side

> Come back to center, extend arms and legs into ...

10

Corpse
At least
5 minutes

Pregnancy

This sequence is designed to help you stay connected to your yoga practice during the physical, mental, and emotional changes of pregnancy. These postures will ease lower back pain, increase strength and flexibility for childbirth, and allow you a wonderful way to de-stress.

1

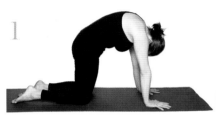

Cat
2 breaths

Exhale into ...

2

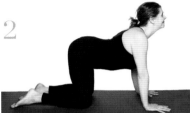

Cow
2 breaths

Release into Tabletop for 3 breaths. Extend into ...

3

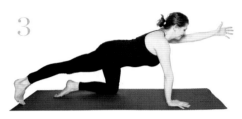

Tabletop, Arm and Leg Variation
3 breaths on each side

Come back to neutral, press back into ...

4

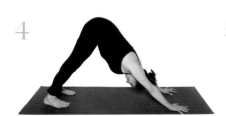

Downward Facing Dog
5 breaths

Walk your hands back to your feet, roll up to ...

5

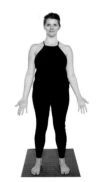

Mountain
3-5 breaths

Exhale into ...

6

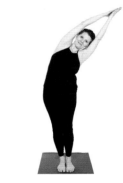

Standing Side Stretch
3 breaths on each side

Come to Mountain, lower into ...

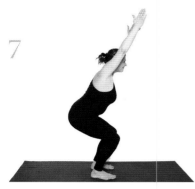

7

Chair
3-5 breaths,
release,
repeat

> Come to Mountain,
> step back into ...

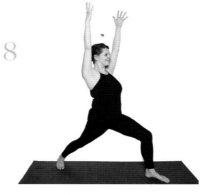

8

Warrior 1
5 breaths

> Open up into ...

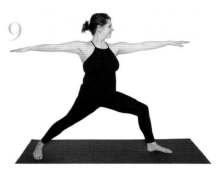

9

Warrior 2
5 breaths

> Repeat Warrior 1 and
> Warrior 2 on the other
> side. Switch back to the
> left side, move into ...

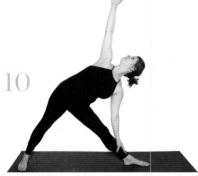

10

Triangle
3-5 breaths
on each side

> Move into Mountain,
> move your feet wide,
> step into ...

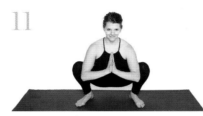

11

Low Squat
5-8 breaths

> Sit on the mat,
> transition into ...

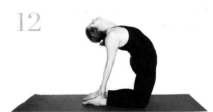

12

Camel
5 breaths

> Plant your hands on
> the mat, move into ...

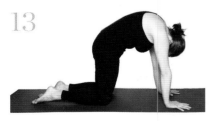

13

Cat
2 breaths

> Exhale into ...

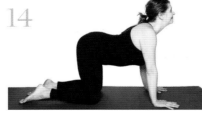

14

Cow
2 breaths

> Sit back on the mat,
> extend your feet
> and move into ...

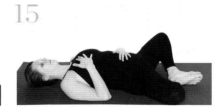

15

Goddess
At least 8
breaths

APPENDIXES

Glossary

ahimsa   Non-harming; a foundational practice in yoga, and the first *yama*.

ananda   Bliss.

aparigraha   Non-hoarding; one of the *yamas*.

asana   Seat, or yoga pose.

ashram   Traditional retreat center, place for spiritual practice.

asteya   Non-stealing; one of the *yamas*.

avidya   Ignorance; the opposite of *vidya*.

Ayurveda   Ancient Indian system of healing and wellness involving using foods, herbs, and the understanding of one's own constitution to achieve balance and health.

Bhakti Yoga   *Bhakti* translates to "devotion" in Sanskrit. Practice is focused on a connection to the divine and often involves chanting and mantra practice as well as a pervasive spiritual bent.

brahmacharya   Responsible use of sexual and creative energy; one of the *yamas*.

chant   A typically repeated phrase sung at a certain limited range of notes. Chanting is sometimes used in yoga practice to calm the mind, open the heart, and connect the yogi to the meaning and tone of the words chanted.

chakras   Translates to "wheel" in Sanskrit and refers to wheels of energy, or energy centers in the body.

chin mudra   Common mudra in which the finger and thumb touch. Typically the thumb gently covers the tip of the finger. With the thumb symbolizing the universe and the finger the individual, this gesture is a reminder of union and protection. Energy is redirected toward these reminders.

dhyana   State of meditation; attention is gently absorbed in one thing.

drishti   Soft yet focused gaze used in yoga practice. Can also refer to a point to focus on, the *drishti* point.

dukkha   Sanskrit term for suffering, stress.

englightenment   Self-realization, realization of interconnectedness of all things. Having the "light turned on" to truth.

gunas   Three qualities or states of being that exist in the universe and in people. They are: *tamas, rajas,* and *sattva*. Different foods, thoughts, and practices can affect these *gunas,* bringing about the different states.

guru   Translates as "dispeller of darkness" in Sanskrit. This term is usually used for a spiritual teacher who guides the student on the path of yoga.

Hatha Yoga   This term refers to the union of dualities. In Sanskrit, *ha* means "sun" and *tha* means "moon." Often the term *Hatha Yoga* is used to describe gentle yoga classes.

inversion   Upside down pose in which the heart is above the head and blood flow is reversed. These poses also allow us to see differently by flipping the view.

japa   The practice of repeating a mantra, often done with mala beads to aid in counting. This practice helps to calm the mind and connect the heart and intentions to that which is being repeated.

karma   Translates to "action" in Sanskrit. In general, the thought is every action has an effect, every seed that is planted brings its own fruits. We can work to plant good seeds.

mantra   A word or phrase repeated with intention. Said to aid the yogi in crossing over from one state of thought to another.

mauna   Silence. A practice in which a yogi keeps silence to better listen within.

maya   Illusion.

mudra   Seal; often shows up in hand positions used in yoga practice.

Namaste   A greeting meaning "the light in me recognizes the light in you."

niyamas   Guidelines for actions and beliefs toward one's self. The *niyamas* are: *saucha*, or "cleanliness;" *santosha*, or "being content and happy with what you have;" *tapas*, or "working hard and with enthusiasm; discipline;" *svadhyaya*, or "studying yourself;" and *ishvara pranidhana*, or "being devoted, or surrendering our efforts to the greater good."

OM   A one syllable *mantra* often used in yoga practice. This sound is considered sacred and represents unity. Many define it as "the sound of the universe."

prana   Life energy, vitality.

pranayama   Breathing exercises.

rajas   A state of agitation or over activity, one of the three *gunas*.

sacrum   A large triangular bone in the lower back, located above the tail bone and in between both hip bones. Sometimes this area is referred to in yoga pose adjustment.

santosha   Contentment.

Sanskrit   Ancient language of India, used often in naming yoga poses and practices and in chanting.

sattva   The state or quality of peace, harmony, and clarity; one of the three *gunas*.

sattvic   Adjective describing things with a state of balance, lightness, and harmony. A *sattvic* diet refers to foods that are gentle and harmonizing to body, mind, and energy.

satya   Truth, truthfulness, honesty; one of the *yamas*.

saucha   Cleanliness; one of the *niyamas*.

savasana   Final resting pose (Corpse Pose).

sukha   Sanskrit term meaning "ease and happiness."

surya namaskar   Sun Salutations; A set *vinyasa*, or flow of poses, made to warm up the body and quiet the mind.

tamas   A quality of sluggishness or heaviness; one of the three *gunas*.

tapas   Discipline or heat; one of the *niyamas*.

ujjayi   "Victorious" breath, often used throughout yoga asana practice.

vinyasa   A flow of poses, one in to the next, with no stopping in between. This practice generates heat in the body, and encourages focus and coordination. We are encouraged to think of transitions just as much as poses themselves in this practice.

vidya   Knowledge; the opposite of *avidya*.

viveka   Discrimination; discerning between the real and unreal.

yamas   Guidelines for one's behavior in the external world and toward others. The *yamas* are: *ahimsa*, or "non-violence; don't do harm;" *satya*, or "honesty; tell the truth;" *asteya*, or "non-stealing;" *brahmacharya*, or "use your creative energy wisely;" and *aparigraha*, or "non-hoarding."

Yoga Sutras   Foundational text of yoga, written down by Patanajali; the *Yoga Sutras* read almost like poems. *Sutra* translates to "thread" in Sanskrit.

yoga   Translates to "union" or "yoke" in Sanskrit. Commonly used to describe a series of practices involving poses, breath work, relaxation, and meditation. Can also refer to a state of being, when one is in harmony and feeling connected.

yogi   A person who practices yoga. Sometimes *yogini* for a female *yogi*.

Resources

Books

There are some wonderful books that can deepen your relationship with yoga. Here are some suggestions, including classic texts like the *Yoga Sutras* and *Bhagavad Gita*. There are also books dealing with specific areas such as chakra study, yoga for kids, mantras, or mudras.

Ashley-Farrand, Thomas. *Healing Mantras: Using Sound Affirmations for Personal Power, Creativity, and Healing.* Wellspring/Ballantine, New York, 1999.

Desikachar, T.K.V. *The Heart of Yoga: Developing a Personal Practice.* Inner Tradition, Rochester, VT, 1995.

Gannon, Sharon and David Life. *Jivamukti Yoga: Practices for Liberating Body and Soul.* Ballantine Books, New York, 2002.

Herrington, Sarah. *OM Schooled.* Addriya, San Marcos, CA, 2012.

Hirschi, Gertrud. *Mudras: Yoga in Your Hands.* Red Wheel/Weiser, York Beach, ME, 2000.

Iyengar, B.K.S. *Light on Yoga: Yoga Dipika.* Schocken, New York, 1966.

Iyengar, B.K.S. *Light on Pranayama: The Yogic Art of Breathing.* The Crossroad Publishing Company, New York, 1985.

Judith, Anodea. *Eastern Body, Western Mind: Psychology and the Chakra System as a Path to the Self.* Celestial Arts, New York, 1996.

Kaminoff, Leslie and Amy Matthews. *Yoga Anatomy, Second Edition.* Human Kinetics, Champaign, IL, 2011.

Lowitz, Leza and Reema Datta. *Sacred Sanskrit Words: For Yoga, Chant and Meditation.* Stone Bridge Press, Berkeley, CA, 2005.

Mitchell, Stephen. *Bhagavad Gita: A New Translation.* Three Rivers Press, New York, 2000.

Mittra, Dharma. *Asanas: 608 Yoga Poses.* New World Library, Novato, CA, 2003.

Myss, Caroline. *Anatomy of the Spirit: The Seven Stages of Power and Healing.* Three Rivers Press, New York, 1996.

Satchidananda, Swami. *The Yoga Sutras of Patanjali.* Integral Yoga Publications, Yogaville, VA, 1978.

Schiffmann, Erich. *Yoga: The Spirit and Practice of Moving into Stillness.* Gallery Books, New York, 1996.

Magazines

To stay up to date in the living conversation of yoga, you may want to check out these magazines which are well respected and have online resources as well as print versions.

Yoga Journal (http://www.yogajournal.com/) is based in San Francisco, California, and is one of the longest-running and most respected yoga magazines.

Yoga International Magazine (http://www.himalayaninstitute.org/yoga-international-magazine/) is published by the Himalayan Institute.

Where to Buy Materials

Luckily yoga has become more popular so it's easy to find yoga mats, clothing, and supplies in stores. Check out sports stores or discount stores in your neighborhood. Here are some places to look online as well, if you're in the market for items for your yoga kit.

Jade Yoga Mats (www.jadeyoga.com) are eco-friendly yoga mats.

Yoga Accessories.com (www.yogaaccessories.com) is a great place to buy mats, blocks, blankets, straps, and cushions individually or in bulk.

Gaiam Online (http://www.gaiam.com) sells not only mats, but yoga clothing and eco-friendly household goods.

Online Learning

If you are interested in learning more about yoga, taking a class, or even becoming certified as a yoga teacher but don't have much available in your area, there are now online options.

YogaGlo (http://www.yogaglo.com) is a directory of videos that can transport you to a class.

Core Strength Vinyasa Yoga Certification (http://www.sadienardini.com/teacher-training.html) allows existing yoga teachers to become trained in this strong, grounded form of yoga.

OM Schooled (www.om-schooled.com) provides complete certification in teaching kids and school-based yoga.

Index

F

fatigue relief, 32-33, 218-219

Fire Log (*Agnistambhasana*), 54-55, 152

Fish (*Maysyasana*), 78-79, 166

flexibility poses

    Cat (*Marjariasana*), 48

    Child's Pose (*Balasana*), 46-47

    Cobra (*Bhujangasana*), 60-61

    Cow (*Bitilasana*), 49

    Cow Face (*Gomukhasana*), 56-57

    Downward Facing Dog (*Adho Mukha Svanasana*), 62-63

    Easy Seat (*Sukhasana*), 40

    Extended Side Angle (*Utthita Parsvakonasana*), 74-75

    Fire Log (*Agnistambhasana*), 54-55

    Fish (*Maysyasana*), 78-79

    Foot Flexion, 42

    Lizard (*Utthan Pristhasana*), 68-69

    Lotus (*Padmasana*), 52-53

    Low Lunge (*Anjaneyasana*), 66-67

    Peaceful Warrior, 72-73

    Pigeon (*Eka Pada Rajakapotasana*), 76-77

    Reverse Warrior, 72-73

    Rock the Baby, 70-71

    Seated Spinal Twist (*Ardha Matsyendrasana*), 50-51

    Shoulder Roll, 44-45

    Standing Side Stretch (*Parsva Tadasana*), 41

    Thread the Needle, 58-59

    Upward Facing Dog (*Urdhva Mukha Svanasana*), 64-65

    Wrist Flexion, 42

Floor Bow, 162

Foot Flexion, 42

G

Garland Pose, 24-25

grounding poses

    Butterfly (*Badhakonasana*), 28-29

    Cobbler's Pose (*Badhakonasana*), 28-29

    Diamond Pose (*Tarasana*), 30-31

    Hero's Pose (*Virasana*), 27

    Low Squat (*Malasana*), 24-25

    Reclining Hero (*Virasana*), 36-37

    Seated One-Leg Forward Fold (*Janu Sirsasana*), 32-33

    Seated Two-Leg Forward Fold (*Paschimottanasana*), 34-35

    Seated Wide Leg Straddle (*Upavistha Konasona*), 22-23

    Staff Pose (*Dandasona*), 26

H

hakini mudra, 205

Half Boat, 164

Half Happy Baby, 129

Half Moon (*Ardha Chandrasana*), 90-91, 163

hands, mudras, 15, 203-205

Happy Baby (*Ananda Balasana*), 130-131

Hatha yoga, vi

headaches, 126-127

Headstand (*Sirsasana*), 196-197

Hear Yourself Think sequence, 228-229

heart *chakra* (*anahata*), 209

Hero's Pose (*Virasana*), 27

High Lunge, 114-115

High Lunge Twist, 154